Go From

TOXIC to TERRIFIC

LEARN HOW TO SURVIVE THE AMERICAN HIGH-TECH DIET

Go From

TOXIC to TERRIFIC

LEARN HOW TO SURVIVE THE AMERICAN HIGH-TECH DIET

Kathryn Parslow

Get Healthy America Publications

Published by Get Healthy America Publications, Puyallup WA
www.HealthTreasureChest.com & www.WaistWatchers.com

We are committed to excellence in the publishing industry. The company reflects the philosophy established by the founders, based on Psalm 68:11,
"The Lord gave the word and great was the company of those who published it."

Book design copyright © 2017 by Get Healthy America Publications. All rights reserved.
Cover design by Amani Hanson

Published in the United States of America
ISBN: 978-1543152531
1. Health and Fitness
2. Diets: Better Health

ACKNOWLEDGMENTS

Writing this book has been one of the most intense experiences of my life. Only at this point in my life has such an undertaking been possible. With children grown and out of the house, and grandchildren out of reach, I've been able to dedicate the time needed to complete this project.

I owe a big, heartfelt thanks to my mentor, adopted mother, inspiration, and dearest of friends, Elizabeth Baker, who passed away peacefully surrounded by friends and family on September 26, 2005. Her oldest son had just read her Psalm 23. Many of her ideas, stories, and writings are included in this book. As a teacher, author and international lecturer, she inspired everyone she met.

To my friend, business partner, visionary, and encourager, I owe so much gratitude. Ron Lowrie has always helped carry the burden of writing, editing and proofing.

To Barbara Randall, PhD—you've been one of the most influential people in my life. Thank you for getting me started in this field of health and nutrition.

To Jonathan Wright, M.D., founder of the Tahoma Clinic in Kent, Washington, thank you for the privilege of working with you. My experiences at the clinic provide a wealth of information and experience to this book.

To Ellouise Carroll, PhD, I greatly appreciate your editing time, your contribution to the book, and your wonderful speaking skills at the Health Treasure Chest Seminars.

This book is very much about preserving the life work of giants in the field. They warned us decades (even centuries) ago that there is a price to pay for ignoring God's natural laws. Forgive us Father and set our feet on a right path.

FOREWORD

By Jonathan V. Wright, MD

Kathryn Parslow's commitment to excellence in nutrition exemplifies one underlying basic rule of her book...."Eat close to nature and you'll reap healthy benefits." It's that simple. Everything you'll read and learn from her book and course enhances and details the why's and why not's of this very simple rule.

The details and scientific explanations will help to convince skeptics that eating whole, natural, unrefined, non-chemicalized food is a key tool for staying healthy!

Have fun with this book. If you're not following all of its principles yet, then very likely your health will improve, from a little to a lot, when you do. It's really not hard. If you think you're getting lost in all the science, or if someone tells you that scientific experts disagree, just refer back to the simple rule above, and you'll get it right, every time!

Jonathan V. Wright M.D.
Tahoma Clinic, Renton, Washington
www.tahoma-clinic.com
Author of *Natural Hormone Replacement for Women Over 45*
and 10 other books about health and nutrition

CONTACT INFORMATION

For information on supplements, herbs, products, food sesitivity testing and equipment, go to www.HealthTreasureChest.com or WaistWatchersWinners.com for more information.

THIS BOOK IS DEDICATED TO PEOPLE EVERYWHERE WHO ARE:

- Sick and tired...
- Worn down by the struggles of twenty-first century life...
- Raising unruly children who are basically good, just out of control...
- Achy, headachy, stiff, and discouraged about it...
- Addicted to alcohol, cigarettes, or some sort of street drug...
- Fed up with buying and taking Rx medications with their host of destructive side effects...
- Nervous, stressed out, and wondering if they are "losing their minds"...
- Diagnosed with a degenerative disease—cancer, heart disease, diabetes...

AND TO PEOPLE EVERYWHERE WHO:

- Want to feel better...
- Want to see their children's behavior and school performance improve...
- Want renewed energy—the energy of their youth...
- Want to be positive, happy, content...
- Want to find a way out of the endless drug and surgery cycle so commonplace today...
- And perhaps want to reach out and help someone else...
- It is our prayer that this book will give you some answers and start you on a new path of renewed health for you and for those you love.

"I will instruct you and teach you in the way you should go"
Psalm 32:8 KJV

TABLE OF CONTENTS

INTRODUCTION

An American Food Dilemma
—Will We Survive?

Hardworking, reliable Bob Johansen has been successful at almost everything he has tried. He was an all American football player, the head of his class in college, and is currently a top notch producer for his company. However, like tens of millions of other Americans—young and old, men and women—Bob is sick. He has a chronic, degenerative disease associated with the American way of life.

In Bob's case, his diagnosis is *metabolic syndrome*. Metabolic syndrome is a cluster of health markers including high cholesterol; high blood pressure; extra weight, particularly around the abdomen; and insulin resistance.[1] When present as a group, the risk for cardiovascular disease and premature death is very high.

Bob has most of these symptoms, including high blood pressure, elevated insulin, a tire of fat around his waist, and high cholesterol. This once healthy, fifty-year-old Washingtonian has just joined the ranks of over 50 million Americans predicted to have metabolic syndrome by 2010. His doctor has told him that major lifestyle changes are in order.

He has been carrying around upwards of an extra 100 pounds for several years and has been planning to go on a diet. For a long time, he knew he was out of control. "The pounds crept on slowly but consistently," he said. "And now I weigh almost 300! My doctor says I am headed for major problems like diabetes, a heart attack, or even worse if I don't do something."

As for exercise, he has pretty much given it up. "I am so heavy that it is hard on my knees to do much at all." He now prefers to watch sports on TV with his teenage children.

A NATION OF FOOD ADDICTS

Like many Americans, Bob has come to favor the convenience and flavor of fast food. He prefers burgers and fries, ice cream, soft drinks, and doughnuts to anything else, eating them all the time—in excess. "I have never cared much about vegetables and prefer the taste of fatty and sweet foods." The Standard American Diet fits right in with Bob's likes. "The energy intensity of the human diet is going up," says Barry Popkin, a professor of nutrition at the University of North Carolina-Chapel Hill. "The most common changes are the added sugar in processed food and the added fat."[2]

Bob has also come to enjoy how convenient it is to eat. "I love how easy it is to get food today. When I was growing up, you had to go to a grocery or drug store to buy a candy bar. Now, you can get a burger and fries and anything else you want on practically every corner in America!" As University of Colorado nutrition researcher James Hill puts it, "Our physiology tells us to eat whenever food is available. And now, food is always available."[3]

MORE FOOD, MORE SICKNESS

Bob is not alone in his struggles. For the most part, the eating habits of our nation have changed dramatically over the last century with the development of sophisticated food-manufacturing technologies and improved agricultural practices. Spurred on by media and advertising hype, we have lost sight of what real food is and assume that anything packaged, tasty, and affordable is well suited to meet our nutritional needs. Unfortunately, such thinking has pushed this nation over the edge of a precipice into a full-blown health crisis.

And thanks to new and better methods of harvesting, transporting, and storing food—coupled with the development of sophisticated fertilizers and pesticides—technology has given us an unprecedented yield of foodstuff per acre, year round.

Judy Putnam, from the USDA, explains that food-supply data shows a 236-calorie-per-person-per-day increase between 1987 and 1994. Between 1994 and 2000, the increase was 500 calories. This averages a 24 pound weight gain per person every year. Putnam figures that about 39% of the increase comes from refined grains, 32% from added fats, and 24% from sugar. The World Health Organization states that in 2016, the daily US calorie intake is 3,770.[4]

BIG FOOD

The food giants are happy to oblige us in filling our dietary wants, regardless of our needs. Also called "big food", here is what Marion Nestle, chair of the Department of Nutrition and Food Studies at New York University, says about these giants:

> Our country has available in the food supply 3,900 calories a day for every man, woman, and child in the country. That's roughly twice what the actual population needs. Food companies are beholden to stockholders. They have to grow in order to maintain their stock prices. We already have 3,900 calories a day and 320,000 different food products in the American marketplace. They can't all keep growing in that situation. So all they can do is to try to get consumers to eat their products instead of somebody else's, or to eat more in general, and they're just terrific at doing that.[5]

It raises the question, have we confused all this lavish quantity and seductive packaging with nutritional riches? Our forebearers had just a few staples—basic foods—on which they relied for centuries. Today in America we have a huge selection of convenience foods all made from these same few basics. However, because of our high-tech processing, these few staples are now severely nutrient deficient.

The World Health Organization recently reported that the U.S. spends a larger proportion of its gross domestic product on healthcare than other countries. So shouldn't we rank number one in health? We don't! In fact, we are only number 37 out of 191 countries in health.[6]

Perhaps it is time we rethink our eating habits and get back to the few basics our ancestors ate—and in their basic form.

DISEASES IN AMERICA

Unlike generations of old where people suffered and died from infectious diseases, modern society has all but eradicated these maladies. We have traded them instead for what has been termed the "diseases of lifestyle." These chronic, degenerative diseases take us down over time. These disorders cause us untold suffering on a daily basis—they may not kill us, but at times they make us wish we were dead!

The statistics are quite astounding. In addition to metabolic syndrome that Bob suffers from, an estimated 652,000 Americans will die of heart disease and 554,000 of cancer this year.[7] Add to that the tens of millions of Americans affected by some form of arthritis, and the nearly 21 million Americans with diabetes.[8] Additionally, millions battle asthma, allergies, and heart or blood-vessel disease.

As for weight issues, Bob isn't alone in his struggle. "More than half of U.S. adults are overweight and millions are obese."[9] Government projections and health providers state that in the next decade, weight-related illnesses will overwhelm the healthcare system.

WHAT HAVE WE DONE TO OUR CHILDREN?

An even more alarming consideration is our children. They, too, are showing the diseases of civilized life including obesity, diabetes, and early signs of heart disease. Overweight levels in children and adolescents have doubled in the last three decades (one in five is currently overweight).[10]

Diabetes, in times past associated only with middle-aged adults, is now prevalent in the youth. A dramatic rise in Type II diabetes is occurring among children with an alarming trend in children as young as six years.

A report from the New England Journal of Medicine concluded that ours might be the first generation to outlive their children stating, "From our analysis of the effect of obesity on longevity, we conclude that the steady rise in life expectancy during the past two centuries may soon come to an end."[11] Quite an alarming and unprecedented thought!

WHAT EXACTLY DO WE EAT?

Eric Schlosser, author of *Fast Food Nation: the Dark Side of the All American Meal*, writes:

> Americans now spend more money on fast food than on higher education, personal computers, computer software, or new cars. They spend more on fast food than on movies, books, magazines, newspapers, videos, and recorded music—combined.[12]

Obviously, junk food consumption has been a major player in our health problems over the last few decades. Comparing 1981 to 2011, the average American consumes in one year:

45 large bags of potato chips—up 78%
120 orders of French fries—up 130%
190 candy bars—up 80%
120 pastries or desserts—up 95%
150 slices of pizza—up 143%[13]

Additionally, estimates are that many Americans eat up to 52 teaspoons of sugar per day, much of it as soft drinks. Actually, "enough soda is produced to supply every American with 1.2 daily 12-ounce drinks, or nearly 200 calories per day from this source alone."[14]

HIGH-TECH PROCESSING & FABRICATION

Until the end of the nineteenth century, the milling of wheat into flour was a rather crude affair involving the use of massive stone wheels that reduced the kernels to a coarse meal. The resulting whole-wheat flour was so nutritionally rich that it was highly perishable and subject to insect and rodent attack.

With the advent of the industrial revolution, a less vulnerable product was wanted. This need was met by new technology, able to completely crush the wheat grain between immense pressure rollers. Then, fine sifting and bleaching yielded the final product—bleached, white flour.

Unfortunately, this grinding and sifting process removes many of the essential food elements that make stone-milled flour so nutritionally viable. Along with the "unsightly" germ, bran, and husk go most of the protein, all of the unsaturated oils, and most of the vitamins and minerals.

Products made from white flour—bread, cakes, cookies, pasta, and bakery goods—have become the mainstay of the American diet. Millions of Americans have no idea that the processing eliminates the nutrients or that there is anything wrong with eating these processed foods on a regular basis.

Not only is white bread devoid of any nutrition (except the five nutrients that are added back after stripping so many of them out), there is a direct correlation between colon and intestinal health and this dietary foodstuff. Fiber helps the colon to be healthier by quickly moving the food through the intestinal system, cleaning it out along the way. With the fiber removed, the food is held in the system long after it should have been expelled. The result is various forms of cancer, one of which is colorectal cancer. "Colorectal cancer causes 50,000 deaths annually and someone dies every 9.3 minutes."[15]

Millions of others suffer from related illnesses such as appendicitis, constipation, colitis, and other intestinal maladies. The simple act of returning to whole-wheat bread and other whole grain products could reduce these statistics dramatically.

Without question, the American food manufacturers have delivered a unique product—a reliable, low-cost food supply. They have supplied foods that will stay "shelf fresh" for months, even years, no refrigeration required, all wrapped up in dazzling packages that captivate the eye. They, too, have given us all the sugar we could ever want in the form of soft drinks, candy, and delectable baked goods that tickle the palate.

But at the heart of the question is the health risks these "manufactured" foods create. Why are we eating "manufactured" foods in the first place? Certainly, our ancestors ate what was natural, organic, whole, basic, and from the earth. Could it be that all these dramatic changes have pushed America into the greatest health crisis of all time?

WHERE DO WE GO FROM HERE?

This brings up the questions: how did we get from there to here? Why do we now need to learn "survival" techniques for something as basic as food? And what can we do about it? Unquestionably, major changes are in order for millions of Americans.

In the meantime, if history has taught us anything, it is that change doesn't happen overnight. It may be decades before we see a major revolution in the food industry and an end to its profiteering from highly processed, denatured, nutrient-devoid, manufactured foods that ultimately can make us sick. And it may take a lot more misery, dying, and many, many more angry Americans willing to raise our voices as a whole, declaring that we've had enough of this national dietary recklessness. Until then—as responsible parents, grandparents, or concerned individuals—it falls squarely on our shoulders. We must take responsibility for our own health by making food choices that will keep us out of harm's way.

A recent report from the Federal Centers for Disease Control and Prevention reported that in 2000, poor diet and obesity, combined with a lack of physical exercise, caused 400,000 deaths, just slightly behind deaths from tobacco. Says Julie Gerbering, Director of the CDC, "It's going to overtake tobacco if this trend continues."[16]

Perhaps it is time for Bob Johansen, and every concerned American, to begin rethinking our dietary choices if we are going to learn *How to Survive the American High-Tech Diet.*

NUTRITION FOR THE MAJOR BODY SYSTEMS

1 The Digestive System

In this section, you'll get an idea of how the food you eat is taken in and utilized by the body. An old adage used by many nutritionally oriented practitioners is that good health begins in the bowels. The theory is that poorly functioning bowels coated with mucous cannot properly absorb the food you eat, no matter how nutritious it is.

Actually, good health begins in the mouth, where digestion starts. First, you must chew your food well (the rule of thumb is twenty to thirty chews before swallowing). Then, your stomach must have adequate *hydrochloric acid* and *digestive enzymes* to properly digest your food. Once

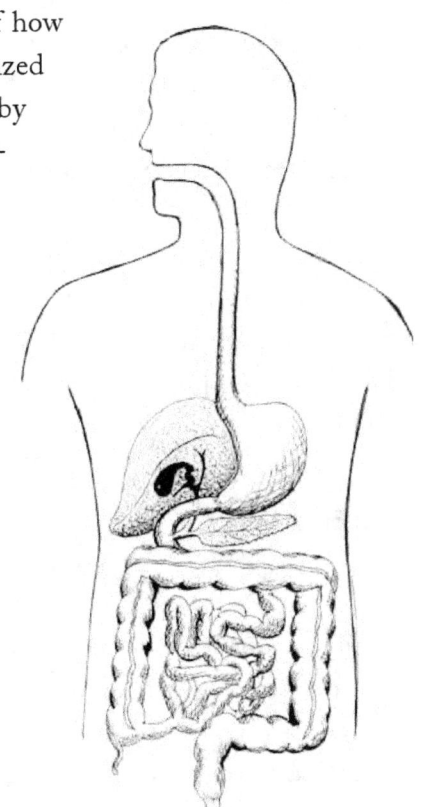

your meal begins its journey through the small and large intestines, what you will actually absorb and metabolize depends on the health of these important organs. Finally, you'll need good elimination to complete the whole process. Think of it as portal-to-portal digestion.

Digestion begins without a single thought on your part. Through a series of automatic chemical and physical changes, your food is broken down and prepared for absorption. Any interruption in this process can cause health issues—from minor stomachaches or gas, to more serious problems like gallbladder disease or even colon cancer.

For a decade, I worked as the clinical nutritionist at the renowned Tahoma Clinic in Kent, Washington, with Jonathan Wright, M.D. It was the learning experience of a lifetime! Dr. Wright emphasized preventive medicine and the use of natural treatments for illness whenever possible. The clinic housed over 35,000 medical journal articles that explained how many symptoms and conditions unresponsive to conventional treatment will yield to the application of nature's remedies.

Many of you may remember Dr. Wright from his 1980s column that appeared in *Prevention* magazine. The majority of the stories in this book are actual experiences I had while working at the clinic. Helen is a case in point. She had a poorly functioning digestive tract and was seeking a natural solution.

HELEN'S STORY

"I HAVE TERRIBLE CONSTIPATION AND STOMACHACHES ALL THE TIME"

Helen Nelson came in to the Tahoma Clinic at the advice of a neighbor who had been a longtime patient of Dr. Wright. Helen had always had bad stomachaches and constipation, but she had become sicker in the past year, and her problems were really starting to affect her work performance. She had missed too much time and felt her job was in jeopardy. She came in to see me after an appointment with Dr. Wright.

"I have terrible constipation and stomachaches all the time. I chew tons of antacids. I've had to miss several days of work just recently, and I simply can't afford to miss any more."

I could see from Dr. Wright's chart notes that she was scheduled for a *Heidelberg Gastrotelemetry stomach acid test*. This simple procedure takes from two to three hours, depending on how much stomach acid the client is producing. During the procedure, a vitamin-sized capsule is swallowed with a string attached to hold it in the stomach. The capsule has a transmitter in it that measures how much stomach acid the patient is producing.

During the test, several sips of bicarbonate are given to neutralize any stomach acid you have. The time it takes for the stomach to re-acidify is measured and charted. Supplemental hydrochloric acid and digestive enzymes are given based on the test results.

"The test sounds painful," she said.

"Sounds like it, I know, but it is really very simple and painless. I've done it myself. Even pulling the capsule back up with the string is easy."

Reading on through Dr. Wright's notes, I could see he had compiled a very thorough history, conducted a complete physical, and had ordered several other tests. He wanted me to talk with her about her highly refined, processed diet.

"Helen, it sounds like Dr. Wright has covered all the bases as far as testing. Let's talk a little about your diet. Tell me what you eat on an average day."

"Well, my diet is rather wretched. I am not a breakfast eater, unless you count the sweet rolls and coffee that I have at about 10:00 in the morning. My lunch is at noon, and I usually take a TV dinner to zap in the microwave. It's something with meat and noodles or rice. Sometimes I take leftover dinner from the night before.

"Dinner is a little more regular. I like packaged dinners with noodles. I add hamburger or tuna."

"Do you eat vegetables or fruits?"

"I have salad occasionally. And I like peas and corn. I do eat apples sometimes, if they are peeled."

"And snacks?"

"I guess its candy or cookies. I like nachos, too."

"Do you drink water, Helen?"

"Usually it's soft drinks or coffee. I might have a glass or two of water a day."

It was easy to see how Helen's diet could be causing constipation. She ate hardly any fiber; most of her food choices were very refined. Even the apple she "sometimes" ate was missing its peel, which is a good source of fiber (and pesticides, too—unless it's organic). And she drank very little water, which is important to keep things flowing smoothly.

I asked her if she knew what dietary fiber was.

"I'm not sure. Isn't it in food that's really bad tasting and hard to swallow?"

"Breads and pastas made with whole grains can be very delicious if you will give them a chance. You are eating mostly processed, devitalized foods that are notoriously lacking in fiber and bulk. They tend to be dry, goopy, pasty, and sticky. They stick to your insides like glue and make evacuation difficult. They just don't do well in making the transit through the bowels," I told her.

"A constant diet like this puts a person on the path of problems like constipation. And in the long run, it sets you up for more serious problems like gallbladder disease or even colon cancer."

"Well, I never heard that from my regular doctor."

"Now that you know, let's figure out what to do about it. We'll start with fiber."

———

A couple of months later, Helen was back in for a follow-up appointment. She had taken very seriously the recommendations that Dr. Wright and I had given her. And she had made major changes to her diet; she was eating mostly whole-grains now and was adding more vegetables and fruits, which she said she "enjoyed sometimes, but ate them whether she wanted to or not."

She also had cut out all the soft drinks and was drinking more water. As I had suggested, she divided her body weight in half, then drank that many ounces of pure water every day (for example, a person weighing 150 pounds should drink at least 75 ounces of water daily).

The hydrochloric acid and digestive enzymes Dr. Wright ordered stopped her stomachaches since her food was now digesting properly.

In my clinical experience, I have seen firsthand that taking unneeded antacids does not improve health; if anything, they make it worse. Antacids stop the flow of hydrochloric acid causing the food to sit in the stomach and ferment. A laboratory test can evaluate the amount of HCl in the stomach. If laboratory testing indicates low or no stomach acid, digestive symptoms usually improve, along with overall health, with the addition of hydrochloric acid and digestive enzymes.

Helen said as she was leaving the clinic on her last visit, "My constipation is gone for the first time in a decade. I had no idea that fiber was so important. Or that digestive enzymes could help so much. I'll never go back to that pasty, white-flour stuff. It feels too good to be regular—I wish I'd known this years ago!"

DIGESTION BEGINS IN THE MOUTH

Digestion begins before the food you are about to eat even enters your mouth; you may smell a delicious meal, or see your favorite pepperoni pizza on a TV ad. Pre-digestion can even begin as you hear food frying or grilling and saliva starts to flow.

Once food enters your mouth, the large pieces are broken down into small particles. The salivary glands produce saliva to moisten food for swallowing and digestion. Enzymes begin the breakdown of carbohydrates in the mouth.

Chewing is one of the most important mechanisms of digestion, yet more often than not is the most forgotten. Chewing is the first stage of digestion. It not only physically breaks down foods, but it signals the organs to secrete their digestive juices (pancreatic enzymes, stomach acids, etc.) in order to prepare for the incoming meal. Try to chew your food until it is a liquid consistency—twenty to thirty chomps!

FOOD ENTERS THE ESOPHAGUS

Once you swallow a mouthful of food, it is no longer under voluntary control. It now passes through the entire body by a process of muscle contractions called *peristalsis*. This automatic action involves a slow, wave-like motion that happens along the entire gastrointestinal tract. Once food has entered your stomach, it is not supposed to slip back into the esophagus (when it does, a condition called *acid reflux* results).

THE STOMACH

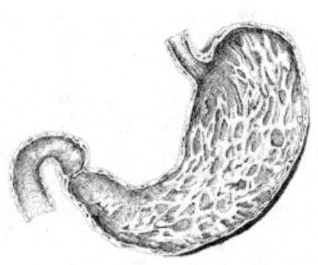

Once in the stomach, the food is mixed with gastric juices containing hydrochloric acid (HCl). HCl is produced by glands in the stomach. It is necessary for the breakdown and digestion of many foods. The stomach's main job is to break down proteins. An enzyme called *pepsin*, combined with HCl, works to do this job.

It takes thirty minutes to six hours, depending upon the foods eaten (less for fruits and vegetables, more for meats), for the peristalsis to push the food, which should now be liquid, out of the stomach and into the small intestine. By this time, the digestion of all three nutrients (proteins, fats, and carbohydrates) has begun. Peristalsis keeps the food moving downward.

THE SMALL INTESTINE & ABSORPTION

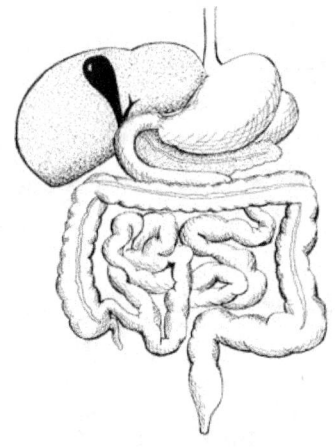

The small intestine is a long tube approximately one inch in diameter and twenty-one feet long. It begins at the stomach and ends where the large intestine begins. Most nutrient absorption happens here through the millions of finger-like projections called *villi*.

When the liquid food enters the small intestine, the pancreas secretes its digestive juices. The food is also acted upon by bile from the liver and gallbladder. By now, your meal is being broken down into body-ready protein, carbohydrates, and fats.

THE VILLI INCREASE ABSORPTION

The villi are hair-like protrusions attached to the inside wall of the small intestine. The purpose of the villi is to slow the passage of food and to allow food particles to be captured in these finger-like protrusions so that the blood can absorb the nutrients in the food.

When the diet is low in fiber, food passes through the intestines slowly, leaving a mucous residue. This results in "mucous-coated" villi that are not able to provide an optimum surface area for good absorption. This lower absorption surface area means less nutrition can be absorbed into the body.

THE LIVER—ORGAN OF DETOXIFICATION

The liver is the only organ that can regenerate itself if parts are damaged. Once food is digested and ready to be absorbed, it passes through the intestinal walls to the liver. The liver secretes bile and acts as a major detoxifier of the body. Many natural health remedies involve liver detoxification.

THE GALLBLADDER

The gallbladder is a three-to-four-inch pear-shaped organ located on the right side of the body just under the liver. The liver produces bile that goes first to the gallbladder where it is held until food arrives in the small intestine. The gallbladder releases the bile, which is ultimately excreted through the colon. Natural gallbladder cleanses concentrate on purging this organ of toxins and gallstones (see index).

THE PANCREAS & DIGESTIVE ENZYMES

A five-to-six-inch long, leaf-shaped organ, the pancreas is situated behind the lower part of the stomach. It has two main functions: to produce digestive enzymes that break down food in the small intestine and to release critical hormones which regulate blood-sugar levels. The pancreas is intimately related to two blood-sugar disorders called *diabetes* and *hypoglycemia* (high and low blood sugar).

THE LARGE INTESTINE OR COLON

The large intestine is the last part of the digestive system. Also called the *colon*, its job is to compact the food residue, absorb water, and produce B-vitamins and vitamin K for healthy intestinal bacteria. Your digestive tract is host to hundreds of different kinds of bacteria (including beneficial, harmful, and neutral types) and yeasts. Among these, *lactobacillus acidophilus* and other members of the lactobacillus family are especially important for the health of your colon.

When the microbial population of the large intestine (also called the gut) is imbalanced, there can be a breeding ground for toxic residue, parasites, and worms. Our Standard American Diet, composed largely of highly refined, white-flour products, does not provide the fiber needed to keep food running smoothly and rapidly through the body. This can lead to many chronic diseases related to poor colon health and habits. Food residues should be eliminated from the body within hours.

Generally, once a meal has been eaten, the previous meal should be eliminated shortly thereafter. This runs quite contrary to the popular idea that eliminating once every three to four days is normal.

ACTION PLAN FOR GOOD DIGESTION
GENERAL RECOMMENDATIONS

- Chew your food well—twenty to thirty chomps per bite, depending on the food. Train yourself not to swallow until the food has turned to a liquid.

- Consume sufficient high-fiber foods daily; these assist the body by producing the "brooming" effect, sweeping clean the intestine.

- Never eat on the run, in the car, or standing at the kitchen counter. Never "shovel in" your meal in a hurry.

- Proper food combining can help with digestion and absorption. As a general rule, do not combine starches (bread, pasta, rice, and potato) with protein (meat, cheese, egg, and fish). Many books are available on the topic of food combining.

- Take the time to make your meals an important and scheduled portion of your day. Mentor and educator, the late Elizabeth Baker always planned each meal hours before she was to eat. Then she set the table with real silverware and china. We live in a society where we grab fast food at the drive through window, unwrap the contents, dig in, and swallow without much chewing.

- Don't consume water or liquids with meals, as they will dilute the hydrochloric acid necessary for digestion. Drink thirty minutes before or sixty minutes after a meal.

DIETARY TIPS

- Beets—Good to detoxify the liver. Take raw, steamed, or added to fresh juice.

- Cabbage—Raw or cooked cabbage contains an obscure nutrient called vitamin U. The U in vitamin U stands for ulcer. Naturopathic physicians claim it is good for peptic and duodenal ulcers. Try freshly squeezed cabbage juice, a few ounces several times a day on an empty stomach.

- Fiber—Replace refined, white-flour foods with whole-grain counterparts to ease constipation.

- Ginger—Excellent as a tea or in food for a stomach calmative.

BENEFICIAL VITAMINS, MINERALS, AND HERBS

Complete Digestive Enzymes—Take these with meals as directed on the label. Professional quality digestive enzymes are available through Metagenics by going to healthtreasurechest.com.

Hydrochloric Acid—Available in pill or capsule, it should be taken only with food. Testing is available to determine if you need this supplement.

Papaya—Has a natural enzyme that aids digestion. Chewable papaya tablets are available in natural food stores.

Pineapple—Contains a natural digestive enzyme called *bromelain* that helps break down food. Bromelain is in many digestive-aid formulas.

Probiotics—Dietary supplements that contain beneficial bacteria such as *acidophilus*. They assist the body's naturally occurring gut flora in proliferating. *Probiotics* are often used after a course of antibiotics or as part of the treatment for gut-related *candidiasis* (yeast overgrowth). Check healthtreasurechest.com for an excellent line of probiotics.

Fresh Vegetables and Fruits—Eat lots of these, with their skins, for fiber. Eat fruit minimally if you have blood-sugar problems.

Water—Divide your body weight in half and drink that many ounces of pure water daily.

GET HEALTHY, AMERICA!

GOOD DIGESTION JUICES

Love Your Liver Tonic
1 small beet
Slice of ginger the size of a quarter
Handful of kale
1 apple

- Push through juicer and drink immediately.

Papaya Pineapple Blast
½ fresh pineapple, including core
1 peeled orange
¼ lemon with peel
1 slice of ginger the size of a quarter
½ papaya

- Push through juicer and drink immediately.

② The Bones

OSTEOPOROSIS: A BONE DISEASE

Complacent is a good word to describe how most people feel about their invisible and boring old bones. Since they are out-of-sight, they are also out-of-mind and of little concern in our daily lives. They've been silently doing a great job of holding us up all our lives. Surely, they'll continue to do so indefinitely...or will they?

Here is an all too familiar scenario: one day in your aging years, you swing a golf club or bend over to pick up your grandchild. *Bam!* You hit the ground! A spontaneous bone fracture has occurred, and a disease that has been progressing slowly and silently but relentlessly rears its ugly head. Jim is a case in point.

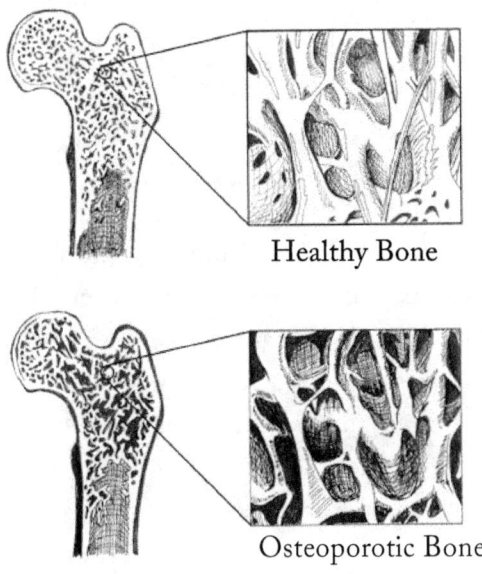

Healthy Bone

Osteoporotic Bone

JIM'S STORY

"I THOUGHT I'D LIVE FOREVER AND NEVER GET SICK"

Jim, a retired aeronautical engineer, was a picture of health. He had a macho physique, a magnificent head of silver hair, and a to-die-for Hollywood smile. At eighty years old, Jim was an active senior citizen with a busy life.

"I felt great and looked great! I thought I'd live forever and never considered getting sick. I had too much life ahead of me."

Jim's home backed up to a beautiful eighteen-hole golf course where he played with his buddies at least three days a week. He also managed all his own yard work and was working on remodeling his family room, with the help of his youngest son.

It was Christmas season, and the kids and grandkids would soon be over for the traditional turkey feast and gift exchange. On the Saturday prior, his wife Ellen asked him to bring down the holiday decorations they kept stored in the attic above the garage.

"I went out to the garage and grabbed a wooden desk chair from the corner. It was a solid, strong chair, and I assumed it would support me. After I retrieved the holiday decorations from the attic, I took a rather hard step backward onto my right foot, and down I went! My foot wasn't the problem. I'd broken my hip."

———

Jim had just joined the ranks of millions who have a silent disease that often makes its presence known only after a light physical task leads to a sudden fracture. It's called *osteoporosis,* and Jim was a victim. "With 1.5 million osteoporosis-related fractures annually, this silent disease poses a serious and growing public health threat."[17]

Literally meaning "holey bones," osteoporosis is a condition where the bones are porous and riddled with holes, much like a sponge.

Osteoporosis occurs more frequently in women than men because female hormones often shut down at menopause, causing a downward shift in the body's ability to absorb calcium, a mineral needed for healthy bones. But it can also affect men, and Jim was one of them. In his own words:

"My quality of life has been dramatically altered. I fear I am on a downhill skid."

OSTEOPOROSIS IN AMERICA: THE STATISTICS

Osteoporosis may progress slowly, or may show up dramatically one day when you take a fall and shatter a hip. Here are some current statistics on osteoporosis from the National Osteoporosis Foundation:

- Osteoporosis is a major public health threat for an estimated 44 million Americans, 55% of whom are fifty years of age and older.

- In the U.S., 10 million individuals are estimated to already have the disease, and almost 34 million more are estimated to have low bone mass, placing them at increased risk for osteoporosis.

- Of the 10 million Americans estimated to have osteoporosis, eight million are women and two million are men.

- Significant risk has been reported in people of all ethnic backgrounds.

- 80% of those affected by osteoporosis are women.

- One in two women and one in four men over the age of fifty will have an osteoporosis-related fracture in her/his remaining lifetime.

- Osteoporosis is responsible for more than 1.5 million fractures annually, including 300,000 hip fractures, 700,000 vertebral fractures, 250,000 wrist fractures, and 300,000 fractures at other sites.

- Women with a hip fracture are at a four-fold greater risk of a second one, and the risk factors are similar to those for the first hip fracture.

- Osteoporotic fractures lower a patient's quality of life.

- The estimated cost (hospitals, nursing homes, and outpatient services) for osteoporotic fractures is $18 billion per year in 2002 dollars, and costs are rising. [18]

OSTEOPOROSIS: WHO IS SUSCEPTIBLE?

The National Osteoporosis Foundation gives some specific markers of those who will get osteoporosis.

Age—The older you are, the greater your risk of osteoporosis. Your bones become weaker and less dense as you age.

Bone Structure and Body Weight—Small-boned and thin women (under 127 pounds) are at greater risk.

Family History and Personal History of Fractures as an Adult—Susceptibility may be due in part to hereditary. Young women whose mothers have a history of vertebral fractures also seem to have reduced bone mass. A personal history that includes a fracture as an adult also increases your fracture risk.

Gender—Your chances of developing osteoporosis are greater if you are a woman. Women have less bone tissue and lose bone more rapidly than men because of the changes involved in menopause.

Lifestyle—Current cigarette smoking, drinking too much alcohol, consuming an inadequate amount of calcium, or getting little or no weight-bearing exercise increases your chances of developing osteo-porosis.

Medications/Chronic Diseases—A significant risk factor is the use of certain medications to treat chronic medical conditions. Rheumatoid arthritis, endocrine disorders (i.e. an under-active thyroid), seizure disorders, and gastrointestinal diseases are treated with medications that may have side effects that can damage bone and lead to osteo-porosis. These medications include glucocorticoids, excessive thyroid hormones, anticonvulsants, antacids containing aluminum, gonado-tropin-releasing hormones (GnRH), methotrexate, cyclosporine A, heparin, and cholestyramine.

Menopause/Menstrual History—Normal or early menopause (brought about naturally or because of surgery) increases risks. Women who stop menstruating before menopause because of con-ditions such as anorexia or bulimia, or because of excessive physical exercise, may also lose bone tissue and develop osteoporosis.

Race—Caucasian and Asian women are more likely to develop osteoporosis. However, African American and Hispanic women are at significant risk for developing the disease.[19]

NUTRIENTS FOR OSTEOPOROSIS PREVENTION

When most people think about building strong bones, they think of getting calcium by drinking milk. While adequate calcium intake is necessary, new evidence suggests that there is more to strong bones than guzzling down the white stuff. Numerous other vitamins and minerals are necessary to help you retain calcium in your bones.

VITAMIN D FOR STRONG BONES

Solid research confirms that a lack of vitamin D is one cause of osteo-porosis. Called the "sunshine vitamin," D is essential for your body to absorb calcium. People who live in sunny climates manufacture more vitamin D than people who live in other climates. Those who live in colder climates are exposed to less sun and are most apt to be vitamin D deficient.

> A recent study found that getting extra high doses of calcium, such as the recommended 1000 milligrams or 1200 milligrams daily, may not be necessary if there is enough vitamin D in the diet. This study from the University of Iceland concludes that "as long as vitamin D status is ensured, calcium intake levels of more than 800 milligrams daily may be unnecessary for maintaining calcium metabolism. Vitamin D supplements are necessary for adequate vitamin D status in northern climates."[20]

As for diet, the following foods have vitamin D: sardines, tuna, milk, and salmon. If you are vegetarian, your diet should include foods that are vitamin D fortified such as some soymilks and ready-to-eat cereals. You can also include broccoli, dandelion greens, figs, hazelnuts, wheat germ, sea vegetables, dark and leafy-green vegetables, soybeans and sesame seeds.

And don't neglect the sunshine; vitamin D is formed when your skin is exposed to the sun. Short exposure—ten to fifteen minutes daily—is enough for most people

VITAMIN K & STRONG BONES

Another cause of osteoporosis is a low intake of vitamin K that is needed for the formation and repair of bones. Dark, leafy-green vegetables such as spinach, kale, collards, and broccoli are good sources of this vitamin. The darker the green, the more vitamin K there is in the food. Other significant dietary sources of vitamin K include beef liver, peas, soybean oil, alfalfa, and green beans. Use dark, leafy-green vegetables in a salad rather than nutrient-deficient iceberg lettuce.

THE MINERAL BORON PREVENTS THINNING BONES

An obscure mineral—*boron*—has been shown to help prevent the thinning of bones that occurs with aging in women. Researchers say that boron dramatically increases blood levels of natural estrogen, a hormone that helps prevent this disease.

An average diet contains about one milligram of boron daily, but up to three milligrams taken as a supplement are shown to be most effective. Good sources of the trace mineral include dates, grapes, beans, raisins, almonds, honey, apples, pears, peaches, peanut butter, soybeans, and hazelnuts. A good defense against osteoporosis is to increase your intake of fruits, nuts, and vegetables.

MANGANESE & OSTEOPOROSIS

Several studies associate a lack of the mineral manganese with severe osteoporosis. The National Research Council's estimated safe and adequate daily dietary intake is two to five milligrams. Higher amounts are often found in high quality vitamin-mineral supplements.

Pineapple is a rich source of the trace mineral manganese, supplying 128% of the amount required daily in just one cup.[21] Other good food sources are pecans, almonds, oatmeal, brown rice, and spinach.

HERBS THAT BUILD STRONG BONES

Alfalfa—Alfalfa roots grow about six feet per year in loose soil.

Metabolically active alfalfa roots have been found sixty feet or more below ground level. The Arabs used alfalfa for their horses, claiming that it made the animals fast and strong. They named the grass "AL-FAL-FA," which means "Father of All Foods." It is relatively high in copper, iron, magnesium, phosphorus, potassium, silicon, sulfur, and zinc. The calcium content is particularly high. Available in tinctures, liquid, tablet, or as an herbal tea, alfalfa contains many minerals that are important for bones, including calcium, magnesium, phosphorus, and potassium.

Horsetail—The herb *horsetail* is a good source of *silica,* a vital component for bone and cartilage formation. It is available in tincture form and as a dried herb. It makes an excellent, mild tea and is a healthy replacement for black tea, coffee, soft drinks, and other sugar-laden beverages. Another name for horsetail is *shavegrass.*

ELIZABETH BAKER'S STORY ABOUT HORSETAIL

"MY BONES LOOKED LIKE SWISS CHEESE"

Our nutritionist, mentor, and friend, Elizabeth Baker, passed away in 2005 at the age of 93. On October 10, 2003, she shared this story at a Get Healthy, America! seminar.

"I had pneumonia in the early summer of 1974. My chest X-rays showed that my bones looked like Swiss cheese from osteoporosis. For many years prior, my nutrition had been poor, as was my digestion and absorption. It wasn't long after that I had the diagnosis of cancer.

"My naturally oriented physician, Dr. Silver, told me about horsetail tea. He said it was the one thing he had used to get patients over osteoporosis. At his advice, I tried the horsetail. I drank a quart of good, strong tea every day. A later X-ray (1980s) of my bones showed they were filled in and as solid as could be.

"For maintenance, I still drink two cups a day—one morning, one evening. I take the tea with my brewer's yeast (brewer's yeast has every known vitamin except B-12 and C). I take the tea straight and strong. It's a mild-tasting herb, but if a person wants to, they can use a little honey or stevia. I advise people nowadays to take a little stevia if they want something sweet."

———

Nettle—A good source of the bone-friendly mineral boron, which helps the bones retain calcium. Nettle makes an excellent herbal tea and is rich in iron, calcium, and various other minerals, especially silica. I was lucky to have a ready source of nettles which grew wild in the woods behind the house my children grew up in. They had learned by trial and error how to pick a nettle without getting stung. I would frequently send them out to harvest nettle, then we would enjoy nettle tea as a family after dinner. As a treat, I'd add a little honey.

Parsley—Rich in vitamins and minerals, including A and C, as well as calcium, thiamin, riboflavin, niacin, zinc, potassium, boron, and iron. Fresh parsley from your grocery store can be used to make tea. Add a sprig to hot water and steep a few minutes as you would regular tea. Rather than leave the decorative parsley on your plate when you eat out, eat it for its health benefits.

BONE-ROBBING CARBONATED BEVERAGES

The latest findings on soft-drink consumption are alarming. Says lead researcher Katherine Tucker, director of the Epidemiology and Dietary Assessment Program at the Jean Mayer USDA Human Nutrition Research Center on Aging at Tufts University:

Among women, cola beverages were associated with lower bone mineral density....Women who drink cola daily had lower bone mineral density than those who drink it only once a week. If you are worried about osteoporosis, it is probably a good idea to switch to another beverage or to limit your cola to occasional use.[22]

Tucker also reported that bone density among women who drank cola daily was almost four percent less than women who did not drink cola, which is significant when you are talking about the density of the skeleton. The effect may be from the caffeine in the cola. Another explanation may have to do with phosphoric acid in cola, which can cause leeching of calcium from bones.[23]

CHILDREN & SOFT DRINKS

The effects of high soft-drink consumption extend beyond women. Michael F. Jacobson, executive director of the Center for Science in the Public Interest (CSPI), said,

Many teens are drowning in soda pop. It's become their main beverage, providing many with 15% to 20% of all their calories and squeezing out more nutritious foods and beverages from their diets. It's time that parents limited their children's soft-drink consumption and demanded that local schools get rid of their soft-drink vending machines, just as they have banished smoking.[24]

Dr. Bess Dawson-Hughes, a bone-disease expert at the Jean Mayer USDA Human Nutrition Research Center on Aging at Tufts University in Boston, said, "I'm particularly concerned about teenage girls. Most girls have inadequate calcium intakes, which makes them candidates for osteoporosis when they're older and may increase their risk for broken bones today."[25]

Writes Carol Simontacchi:
Americans drank twice as many soft drinks in 1997 as they did in 1973, and forty-three percent more than in 1985. Americans gulp twice as much soda as milk and nearly six times more soda than fruit juice. Manufacturers produce enough pop to provide every American with fifty-four gallons per year.[26]

Since our children need to form strong bones in their youth, removing soda pop from their diets is a good idea.

EXERCISE FREQUENTLY & HABITUALLY

Bones are living tissue that respond to exercise by becoming stronger and denser the more they are used. The National Osteoporosis Foundation says,

You cannot see your bones respond to exercise, but when you strike a tennis ball or land on your feet after jumping, chemical messengers tell your arm and leg bones to be ready to handle that weight and impact again. In fact, if you X-rayed the arms of a tennis player, you would see that the bones in the playing arm are bigger and denser than the bones in the other arm.

Two kinds of exercise are important: weight-bearing and resistance exercises. Weight-bearing exercises are exercises that work against gravity like jogging, walking, stair climbing, or dancing. The second type of exercise is resistance exercise, which includes activities that use muscular strength, activities like weight lifting (using free weights or dumb bells, and/or weight machines found at gyms and health clubs).

The National Osteoporosis Foundation further says,

Most weight-bearing and resistance exercises place health demands on bone. Daily activities and most sports involve a combination of these two types of exercises. An active lifestyle filled with varied physical activities strengthens muscles and improves bone strength.[27]

ACTION PLAN FOR HEALTHY BONES & JOINTS
GENERAL RECOMMENDATIONS

- Follow a whole, natural diet rich in the bone-friendly nutrients listed below. People with osteoporosis should achieve their ideal weight through diet modification and a healthy exercise program.

- Smoking, alcohol consumption, and excessive salt intake should be greatly reduced.

- To avoid the need for *acid-blocking drugs (PPI therapy)*, eat smaller meals and avoid coffee, citrus juices, soda, alcohol, fatty foods, and hot spices. A report published in the Journal of the American Medical Association said that, "long-term PPI therapy, particularly at high doses, is associated with an increased risk of hip fracture."[28] Proton Pump Inhibitors (PPI) include Aciphex, Nexium, Prevacid, Prilosec, and Protonix.[29]

DIETARY TIPS

- Buy fresh grapes and freeze a serving size in individual bags. Called "grape-pops," they will always be available, make a great between-meal snack, and are rich in boron.

- Consume kale, parsley, spinach, or oranges for vitamin C.

- Dark, leafy-green vegetables are good sources of bone-friendly minerals. Replace common iceberg lettuce salads with these greens.

- Drink unsweetened pineapple juice for a snack instead of a soft drink.

- Eat pineapple for manganese, which strengthens bones.

- Significantly reduce your consumption of coffee, soft drinks, and alcohol.

- Sprinkle sesame seeds on salads for extra calcium.

- Use ginger, apples, dates, and pears for boron.

BENEFICIAL VITAMINS, MINERALS, AND HERBS

The following nutrients are beneficial. Visit healthtreasurechest.com for a high quality bone-supporting supplement.

Boron—Helps stop bones from thinning due to hormone/menopause symptoms.

Calcium—Keeps bones hard and strong. Excellent sources are bok choy, broccoli, collards, kale, mustard greens, and turnip greens. Sardines and salmon canned with bones are also good sources.

Vitamin D—Helps the body properly use calcium and phosphorus.

Magnesium—Activates enzymes that help form new calcium crystals.

Manganese—Helps build bone and cartridge.

Vitamin C—Essential for building collagen, the protein that forms the underlying bone-matrix.

Vitamin K—Aids the supporting structure, which helps hold calcium in bones.

GET HEALTHY, AMERCA!

BONE-BUILDING JUICES

Calcium-Rich Beverage
  Handful of spinach
  1 slice ginger the size of a quarter
  Handful of kale
  1 apple
  1 spear fresh pineapple

- Bunch up kale and spinach. Push through juicer. Follow with pineapple, apple, and ginger. Drink immediately.

Manganese Mania Juice
  ½ fresh pineapple, including core
  ¼ peeled lemon
  1 slice ginger the size of a quarter

- Push through juicer. Drink immediately.

3 Arthritis—A Joint Disease

Arthritis, a painful condition involving the joints, is a multi-million dollar disease. "More than 55 million Americans suffer from osteo-arthritis, rheumatoid arthritis, and related conditions."[30] There are dozens of different kinds of arthritis. Two of the most common are *osteoarthritis* and *rheumatoid arthritis.*

Osteoarthritis is a disease of the joints resulting in stiffness, pain, and a limited range of motion. This form of arthritis usually doesn't develop before the age of forty, but it affects millions over the age of sixty. The disease causes the joints to dry out as they do not receive needed fluid and nutrition.

Rheumatoid arthritis is a type of inflammatory arthritis. It is a self-attacking-self disease that creates stiffness, swelling, fatigue, and often crippling pain. Over two million Americans have this disabling disorder, the majority of which are female. It can even strike children under the age of sixteen.

ACTION PLAN FOR ARTHRITIS RELIEF
GENERAL RECOMMENDATIONS

- While the cause of arthritis is not completely understood, it is thought to be related to the immune system (*autoimmunity*), a poor diet with too much sugar and meat, and a lack of nutri-ent-rich fruits and vegetables. Arthritis can be slowed and even reversed in some cases by lifestyle and dietary changes.

DIETARY TIPS

- Follow a basic whole-food, natural, fiber-rich, and nutrient-dense diet plan. A vegetarian diet may be beneficial, particularly one rich in raw foods.

- For all arthritic conditions, it may be very beneficial to check for food allergy/sensitivities. See the Food Sensitivity Test Tab at healthtreasurechest.com.

- New studies find that tart, red cherries can relieve arthritic pain— eat up to twenty daily.

- Nightshade foods have long been associated with causing arthritic pain. The family includes tomatoes, potatoes, eggplant, peppers, and tobacco.

- Pineapple is a good source of bromelain, an enzyme that helps reduce inflammation. Available in capsules; take between meals.

- Since sulfur is used for rebuilding bone and cartilage, eat more sulfur-containing foods: eggs, garlic, onion, and asparagus.

- Stretching and strengthening exercise is important to slow or reverse arthritis. Check with your healthcare practitioner first.

- Drinking green tea may be beneficial. In a recent study at the University of Michigan Medical School, scientists found that ingredients in the tea could inhibit several molecules involved in inflammation and joint damage of rheumatoid arthritis.[31]

BENEFICIAL VITAMINS, MINERALS, AND HERBS

Also beneficial and found in arthritic-support supplements— Boron, calcium, silica, sea cucumber, and vitamin K.

Essential Fatty Acids (omega-3 and omega-6)— Taken as directed on label, help reduce inflammation.

Glucosamine Sulfate and **Chondroitin Sulfate**— Are two nutrients that support joints and bones. Take as directed on label.

MSM (*methylsulfonylmethane*)— A sulfur compound used to reduce inflammation, supports connective tissue that is destroyed as part of the disease (MSM should not be taken by sulfur-sensitive people).

Herbs—Alfalfa, Cat's Claw, Green Tea, Cayenne, Nettle, and Willow Bark are helpful as teas, tinctures, or capsules.

Vitamin C— Helps prevent joint swelling.

GET HEALTHY, AMERICA!

ARTHRITIS FRESH JUICE

Aches-Away Delight
 1 handful parsley
 2 stalks celery
 1 apple
 1 slice ginger the size of a quarter

•   Push through juicer and drink immediately.

4 The Brain and Nerves

For decades, we've heard that high blood pressure and elevated cholesterol are dangerous because they put us at risk for having a heart attack. Massive advertising campaigns were launched in an effort to get us to reduce fat, eat more fruits and vegetables, exercise, and reduce stress. Unfortunately, we were never told that similar choices could keep our brains healthy well into old age.

Recently, there has been a dramatic shift, and researchers now say that by giving our brain the nutrition it needs, we can ultimately determine how well it will function as we age. They say that taking action now can slow or halt brain diseases of all kinds. It's all part of the revolutionary natural health movement that stresses prevention, not just treatment after we are sick. It's good to know that nutritional and lifestyle choices can ultimately improve our brain and even save us from the dreaded mental diseases of our time.

THE WORK OF THE BRAIN & NERVES

The brain and nervous system are your body's main control centers. Their jobs are to sense changes in the body, to interpret those changes, and to respond with muscular contractions or glandular secretions. In just a split-second, the nerves can make the needed adjustments to keep your body functioning efficiently.

Your body produces *neurotransmitters*, which are brain chemicals that act like electrical switches. These neurotransmitters are ultimately responsible for all the functions of the body. When there is reduced production of them or a lack of the nutrients from which to make them, your brain will develop the equivalent of a power failure or a short circuit.[32]

VITAMINS & MINERALS BUILD NEUROTRANSMITTERS

We know that food can have a tremendous effect on diseases such as cancer, arthritis, and heart disease—the lifestyle diseases of Western society. But now, scientists are showing that food can also impact the brain and memory.

Pioneering new research documented in numerous studies shows that what you eat can determine your alertness, your mood, your memory, and even your susceptibility to a whole list of neurological diseases from schizophrenia to Alzheimer's disease. The mineral boron is just one example. In a study on this mineral, the importance of nutrients for brain function was demonstrated.

Researcher James Penland, PhD, found that not getting enough boron in the diet can slow your mental alertness. In his studies, he put healthy older men and women on high or low boron diets. The people who were eating less boron had slow electrical activity in their brains. When their diets were extremely deficient in boron, performance on menial tasks decreased even more.

> They could not tap their fingers as fast or pick out specific letters of the alphabet as quickly. The bottom line: they were just not as alert. But when they went on a high-boron diet, their brainwave activity picked up.[33]

Boron is found in nuts, legumes, dark and leafy-green vegetables, broccoli, fruits, dates, apples, pears, peaches, and grapes. Boron is simply one example of the power of food on the brain. Hundreds of research studies confirm—and reconfirm—that foods of all kinds can affect the function of the brain, positively or negatively. Because nutrients are critical for proper function, it is imperative that the diet be rich in whole, unrefined, and nutrient-dense foods.

THE BRAIN & ALZHEIMER'S DISEASE

Alzheimer's is a type of *dementia*, a decline of mental function. It is named for Aloysius Alzheimer (1864–1915), a German psychiatrist with the first published case of pre-senile dementia, which would later be called Alzheimer's disease. It was in the early 1900s that Dr. Alzheimer noticed a patient with strange behavioral symptoms, including loss of short-term memory. This patient became his obsession, and he studied her for years.

Estimates are that up to 5.1 million Americans suffer from Alzheimer's disease (AD). The disease usually begins after age 60, with risks increasing as age goes up. About five percent of men and women ages 65 to 74 have AD. However, it is not a reality of aging.[34]

This is an alarming statistic once you consider the U.S. Census Bureau report that in 2006, the oldest of the baby boomers turned 60; as of mid-July 2005, there were 78.2 million baby boomers over 60; 7,918 people are turning 60 each day, equaling 330 every hour.[35]

Again, nutrition comes in to play. While the causes of Alzheimer's are not entirely understood, research points to many clues, including nutritional deficiencies. Some studies indicate that a lack of adequate vitamin B-12 and zinc may be associated with the onset. It is known that B vitamins are important for proper cognitive functioning. Our modern and highly processed junk foods have been stripped of most of their B vitamins.

IS THERE AN ALZHEIMER'S–ALUMINUM CONNECTION?

Another generally unnoticed but certainly important risk factor for developing Alzheimer's is exposure to aluminum. While the theory is considered controversial, manufacturers have picked up on the potential problem, offering everything from aluminum-free antiperspirants and shampoo to aluminum-free antacids.

Scientific studies on the connection between Alzheimer's and aluminum have appeared in highly respected medical journals. Michael A. Weiner, executive director of the Alzheimer's Research Institute writes:

> Aluminum has been known as a *neurotoxic* substance for nearly a century. The scientific literature on its toxic effects has now grown to a critical mass. It is not necessary to conclude that aluminum causes Alzheimer's disease to recommend that it be reduced or eliminated as a potential risk. It is the only element noted to accumulate in the tangle-bearing neurons characteristic of the disease and is also found in elevated amounts in four regions of the brain of Alzheimer's patients.[36]

It just makes good sense to avoid aluminum products as much as possible. This would include antiperspirants (read label), aluminum cans, cookware, foil, over-the-counter painkillers, douche preparations, baking powders, toothpaste, bleached flour, grated cheese, table salt, and beverages packaged in aluminum cans. Choose more natural options: beverages in glass bottles, natural deodorants and toothpastes, aluminum-free baking powder, and glass bowls with glass lids. Check out your local natural food store for these items.

A WORD ON MERCURY & ALZHEIMER'S

Another controversial subject is the health problems associated with mercury. In his book, *Health and Nutrition Secrets that Can Save Your Life,* Russell Blaylock, M.D., has a chapter called "Mercury, the Silent Killer." For anyone interested in this topic, you will find his book very informative (as well as his book *Excitotoxins, the Taste the Kills*). He writes that there is growing evidence that low-level chronic mercury exposure is associated with numerous disorders, including multiple sclerosis, Alzheimer's, Dementia, Parkinson's disease, and ALS.[37]

And Dr. James Balch writes:

> Brains of people with Alzheimer's disease have been found to contain higher than normal concentrations of the toxic metal mercury. For most people, the release of mercury from dental amalgams is the primary means of mercury exposure, and a direct correlation has been demonstrated between the amount of inorganic mercury in the brain and the number of amalgam surfaces in the mouth. Mercury from dental amalgam passes into body tissues, and it accumulates in the body over time. Mercury exposure, especially from dental amalgams, cannot be excluded as a major contributor to Alzheimer's disease.[38]

ADDICTIONS & THE BRAIN

Addiction is a chronically relapsing brain disease. Brain imaging shows that addiction severely alters areas in the brain critical to decision-making, learning, memory, and behavior control, which may help to explain the compulsive and destructive behaviors of addiction. The National Institute on Drug Abuse explains the addictive process as follows:

Some drugs work in the brain because they have a similar size and shape as natural neurotransmitters. In the brain in the right amount or dose, these drugs lock into receptors and start an unnatural chain reaction of electrical charges, causing neurons to release large amounts of their own neurotransmitter. Some drugs lock onto the neuron and act like a pump, so the neuron releases more neurotransmitters. Other drugs block re-absorption or reuptake and cause unnatural floods of neurotransmitters. All drugs of abuse, such as nicotine, cocaine, and marijuana, primarily affect the brain's limbic system. Scientists call this the "reward" system. Normally, the limbic system responds to pleasurable experiences by releasing the neurotransmitter dopamine, which creates feelings of pleasure.[39]

There are many excellent treatment plans, treatment centers, books, and other resources to help anyone with addiction issues. Since this book is about nutrition, we will focus on what can be done to help an addictive personality by using nutritional methods. Marion found help from reading *The Missing Diagnosis*.

MARION'S STORY

"I WAS HANGING BY A VERY FINE THREAD"

"As a chronic alcoholic, I entered a traditional treatment program. Although some of it was extremely helpful, it failed to help me with the intense confusion, irritability, depression, anxiety, and nervousness that I continued to have, putting me at high risk of relapsing.

After a year of untold suffering and "white knuckling" it, I was left hanging by a very fine thread. I attended an AA meeting every day and was an active participant, working the program as I had been instructed.

One day, a friend gave me the book *The Missing Diagnosis* by Dr. Orion Truss. It changed my life! I needed to find a doctor familiar with these protocols, so I was fortunate to get an appointment with the eminent Dr. Jonathan Wright at the Tahoma Clinic in Washington state. He was knowledgeable in alternative approaches to alcoholism. He tested me for food allergies, chemical allergies, hypoglycemia, and vitamin and mineral deficiencies.

It was when I addressed these issues that I finally found something to change my life and give me control of my urge to drink. I discovered that by eliminating sugar and wheat from my diet, I could also eliminate my disabling anxiety and depression. By identifying and eliminating all the foods I was sensitive to, along with addressing my hypoglycemia and nutritional deficiencies, I turned my mental health completely around. I was soon no longer "white knuckling" it to stay sober. I've been sober for twelve years now without the necessity of attending AA meetings. Best of all, I don't have cravings for alcohol or any other substance."

ACTION PLAN FOR A HEALTHY BRAIN
GENERAL RECOMMENDATIONS

- Eat a well-balanced diet of whole, natural foods with plenty of raw fruits and vegetables. Include foods rich in antioxidants everyday. Those highest in antioxidants are brightly colored produce—apples with skins, prunes, cherries, berries of all kinds, vegetables (particularly dark, leafy-green vegetables), nuts, and seeds. Avoid anything with chemical additives, preservatives, and artificial colors and flavors.

- For good memory and Alzheimer's prevention, keep yourself active mentally by using your brain daily on such things as reading, crossword puzzles, learning a new language, or learning to play a new instrument. Learning a new language or learning to play an instrument exercises both the right and left side of the brain, which is very beneficial.

- It may be helpful to have testing done to rule out any food allergies. Numerous researchers note that reactions to common foods can cause headache, depression, confusion, and other mental aberrations. Several very common trigger foods are wheat, milk, corn, eggs, and soy.

- Studies have also indicated that hypertension, high cholesterol, the presence of too much *homocysteine* in the blood and smoking are potentially important risk factors for Alzheimer's disease.[40]

- Getting oxygen to the brain through deep breathing and exercise is also essential.

DIETARY TIPS

- High-quality protein foods provide amino acids to build *neurotransmitters*. Include in the diet: natural eggs, cheese, lean cuts of meat, turkey, and chicken. Vegetarian sources of protein include nuts, seeds, and soy protein.

- Recent research has shown the importance of essential fatty acids (EFA's) for normal mood and brain function. EFA's are found in wheat germ, walnuts, dark and leafy-green vegetables, seeds, some fish, and flaxseed. These foods should be a regular part of a brain-healthy diet.

- Using *lecithin*, a major source of *choline*, may be beneficial. Choline is a precursor (forerunner) of acetylcholine, a brain chemical essential for a smooth flow of nerve impulses. Choline is found in egg yolks, lecithin, meat, and soybeans. Granulated lecithin is available in natural food stores and makes a good addition to smoothies.

BENEFICIAL VITAMINS, MINERALS, AND HERBS

Low Thiamine (B-1)— Levels are linked to some impairments in brain activity. Known as the nerve vitamin, it is concentrated in wheat germ, bran, nuts, meat, and whole-grain cereals.

Selenium— Researchers at University College in Swansea, Wales, gave people either 100 micrograms of selenium a day or a placebo for five weeks. After a few months, they switched the people to the opposite pill. Moods improved markedly when the patients were taking the selenium.[41] Selenium is found in whole grains, garlic, meat, seafood, and Brazil nuts.

The **B Vitamins**— Are important for brain function. Processed foods are notoriously deficient in these vitamins.

GET HEALTHY, AMERICA!

BRAIN-BUILDING JUICE

Memory Maker
  1 handful each: kale, spinach, romaine, collard greens
  1 apple

• Push through juicer and drink immediately.

5 The Cardiovascular System

It begins in childhood and progresses silently and slowly as plaque starts to form in your arteries. Then one day later in life, the stiff, hard stuff that's been piling up sends the dreaded signal to your body—heart attack! Your loved one runs for the phone and dials 911. Paramedics burst through the door and begin life-saving procedures. This time, the attack has been caught in time and not too much damage has been done. My mother-in-law Alice was one of the lucky ones.

ALICE'S STORY

"I FELT LIKE AN ELEPHANT WAS SITTING ON MY CHEST"

Alice was fifty-nine years old and seemed to be in great health. She seldom had headaches, colds, or the flu. Energy was never a problem for Alice; she always had plenty of it when it came time to babysit the grandkids. She loved life and lived it to the fullest.

Alice was always doing some sort of a project, seeming to never stop, except in the evenings when she would put on her robe and grab a good novel. Busy as she was, most of her activities took place while she was sitting down—painting, making ceramics, quilting, or working on her needlepoint. Like most people of that generation, she never walked, jogged, or did any activity that would raise her heart rate.

As for diet, Alice only liked certain foods—very specific foods. She figured that food was to be enjoyed and always said, "I don't like vegetables and fruits. Just give me meat and potatoes, and lots of gravy. And let me have my tea—strong and sweet."

She would habitually drink three or four cups of black tea a day, with sugar—tons of sugar! She would tilt the sugar container toward her cup and let it flow. Then she'd put a teaspoon under the stream and measure four spoonsful. Everyone knew it was far more sugar than that, but she was so defensive about it that we stopped saying a word.

One evening late, she awoke to an excruciating pain in her jaw and left arm. She slipped into her robe and went to the kitchen, where she put the tea water on. Something was terribly wrong, and she knew it.

She told us later, "I felt like an elephant was sitting on my chest. I was sure I was having a heart attack. I yelled for Del, and he came quickly. The next thing I remember, I was speeding down the freeway in the back of an ambulance."

Alice had had a heart attack. Her arteries were severely blocked and open-heart surgery was scheduled immediately.

Considering the fact that 250,000 people die of heart attacks each year before they reach a hospital,[42] my mother-in-law was indeed, one of the lucky ones. Her surgery was successful, and she lived another twenty-two years. Those years saw some serious dietary and lifestyle changes; no more smoking, very little sugar (which meant no more tea since she really drank it for the sugar), and daily exercise.

As she said a few months later: "It was the scare of a lifetime. I guess it took that to get my attention. I am so grateful for the years I've been given and the chance to see my grandkids grow up."

STATISTICS ON HEART DISEASE

Cardiovascular disease is a term used for heart attack, stroke, and other heart and blood-vessel disorders. Also called heart disease, it is the number one cause of death in the United States, claiming more than one million lives annually.[43] Nearly 801,000 people in the United

States died from heart disease, stroke, and other cardiovascular diseases in 2013. That's about one of every three deaths in America. Many do not know it because they have no symptoms.

"Traditionally thought to be a disease primarily affecting men, it is also increasingly a problem for women. In 2004, 461,152 American females died from CVD, and 7.2 million females had coronary heart disease (CHD)." [44]

SOME COMMON CIRCULATORY DISORDERS

Angina: Angina occurs when the heart gets too little blood. Chest pain, pressure, or a squeezing pain is one sign of angina. The pain could also be in the shoulders, jaw, and sometimes in the back or arms.

Arteriosclerosis/Atherosclerosis: Also called hardening of the arteries. The two forms include a gradual calcium deposit in the artery walls (arteriosclerosis) and the more serious atherosclerosis, a buildup of calcium along with cholesterol and fatty deposits in the artery walls.

Blood Clot: A clot forms when clotting factors in the blood cause it to coagulate or become a solid, jelly-like mass. When a blood clot forms inside a blood vessel, it can dislodge and travel through the blood stream, causing a heart attack or stroke.

Heart Attack: When blood flow to a portion of the heart is blocked, a heart attack occurs. Since blood carries oxygen to the heart, if the flow isn't rapidly restored, that portion of the heart becomes damaged and begins to die from oxygen depletion.

High Blood Pressure (Hypertension): As the heart pumps blood into the arteries, the blood flows with a force pushing against the walls of the arteries. Blood pressure is the product of the flow of blood times the resistance in the blood vessels. High blood pressure is also called hypertension. What makes high blood pressure important is that initially it may cause no symptoms but can still cause serious long–term complications.[45]

Stroke: When blood supply to the brain is cut off, brain cells die from lack of oxygen and other nutrients. Some symptoms include inability to speak, tingling in the limbs, loss of movement in the limbs, and/or impaired memory. This may occur when a clot is formed, which then interrupts the blood flow to the brain. Usually, the result is neurological damage.

ACTION PLAN FOR A HEALTHY HEART
GENERAL SUGGESTIONS

- The dietary, nutritional, and lifestyle recommendations listed here are designed to help prevent you from having a heart attack and to give your cardiovascular system the best possible nutrition. *They are not meant for emergency treatment. If you ever think you may be having a heart attack, seek medical assistance immediately.*

- Follow a natural, whole-food plan with lots of fruits and vegetables. Incorporate plenty of dark, leafy-green vegetables for their nutrient and chlorophyll content. Replace sugary snacks with raw nuts and foods rich in magnesium and potassium (see dietary tips). It is never too early or too late to make these changes.

- You can take a simple, home pulse test to forewarn of oncoming illness. First thing in the morning, place the first two fingers of your right hand between the bone and the tendon of your left wrist. Count the beats for fifteen seconds and then multiply by four. The rate should be 60 to 100 beats per minute.

- Watch your iron levels if you are a woman. University of Florida researcher Jerome Sullivan, M.D., explains that each time you give blood, you remove some of the iron it contains. High blood iron levels, Sullivan believes, can increase the risk of heart disease. Iron has been shown to speed the oxidation of cholesterol, a process thought to increase the damage to arteries leading to cardiovascular disease.[46]

DIETARY TIPS

- B Complex-Rich Foods— B-6, B-3 and folic acid deficiencies are linked to heart disease. The American diet is very deficient in the B vitamins, which are found in dark, leafy-green vegetables and whole grains.

- Buckwheat— Asian countries use noodles made from buckwheat flour (soba). Buckwheat is a non-gluten grain used to make pancakes, breads, noodles, and muffins. Diets that contain buckwheat are linked to lowered risk of developing cardiovascular disease. Buckwheat's beneficial effects are due in part to its rich supply of health-giving flavonoids, particularly rutin.

- Chocolate— Some new studies are showing that dark chocolate has antioxidant properties and reduces blood clotting. The chemical in cocoa beans has a biochemical effect similar to aspirin. But keep in mind that the high sugar and fat of chocolate can cancel out most of these benefits.

- Cold Water Fish— Because fish is packed with important omega-3 fatty acids, fish eaters worldwide have less heart disease. Just two to three servings of fish a week may protect against stroke and heart problems.

- Fiber— A study published in the Archives of Internal Medicine confirms that eating high fiber foods like apples helps prevent heart disease."[47] Simply put, eat whole foods with all their components intact.

- Garlic and Onions— Literally hundreds of studies have been done on garlic and onions attesting to their healthful benefits. They both have heart protective sulfur compounds and the antioxidant quercetin.

- Other Heart-Friendly Foods— Hot peppers, black mushrooms, ginger, cloves, all vegetables, olive oil, tea, and red wine (in moderate amounts).

- Homocysteine— Homocysteine is an amino acid produced by the body, but studies suggest high levels are associated with increased risks of cardiovascular disease. While homocysteine has necessary functions in the body, a deficiency of folic acid, B-6 and B-12 can retard its proper breakdown. Foods rich in these B vitamins are okra, orange juice, potato, banana, and salmon.

- Magnesium-Rich Foods— Magnesium is found in whole-wheat, nuts, dairy, apples, avocados, black-eyed peas, grapefruit, and dark and leafy-green vegetables. Magnesium and potassium are two minerals that are important for the contraction and relaxation of the heart. Potassium-rich foods are apples, avocados, carrots, broccoli, sunflower seeds, oranges, peanut butter, bananas, brewer's yeast, tomatoes, and salmon.

- Natto— Natto is a traditional Japanese food commonly eaten for breakfast in Japan. Made from soybeans fermented by Natto bacillus, it is sticky and strong smelling and tasting. Natto contains a fibrinolytic enzyme called *nattokinase*. It is reported to reduce and prevent blood clots, heart attacks, and strokes. It is readily available in Asian food stores. Nattokinase is also available in capsules. It may interfere with some drugs, so take it under medical supervision.

- Raw Nuts— Raw nuts have all been shown to be heart protective in numerous studies. In the landmark Seventh Day Adventist study on over 31,000 people, it was found that those who ate nuts five times a week had half the chance of heart attack and coronary death.[48] Nuts are rich in antioxidants, vitamin E, selenium, and other phytochemicals. But hold the salted, oiled, and baked nuts. They won't give you the same protection as nuts fresh from the shell.

BENEFICIAL VITAMINS, MINERALS, AND HERBS

Carnitine— This is a substance resembling an amino acid but related to the B vitamins. It improves oxygen uptake and helps prevent fatty buildup in the heart. It is found mainly in red meat and dairy products, but small amounts are contained in whole-wheat bread and asparagus.

Cayenne— In *Left for Dead*, author Dick Quinn describes his miraculous improvement from a failed heart surgery with the herb cayenne. Cayenne has been used historically as a blood thinner and to increase blood circulation. Dick Quinn's book is available on the internet.

Coenzyme Q10—*CO-Q10* is a strong antioxidant described as "vitamin-like." It is present in all cells of the body. Known as a heart re-energizer, it increases oxygen to the heart as documented in numerous studies.

Essential Fatty Acids— These fatty acids are heart protective. Rich sources are nuts, seeds, and cold water fish.

Ginkgo Biloba— This is an herb with powerful antioxidant effects on the cardiovascular system. It may have drug interactions, so use it under a doctor's direction. Available in capsules or tinctures.

Hawthorne Berry— Widely used as a heart tonic, particularly in Europe. It can be used to help regulate blood pressure and break down cholesterol and fat that may contribute to heart disease. It is available in natural food stores, in capsules, tinctures, or tea.

OPC (Oligomeric Procyanidins)— These nutrients are derived from grape seeds and the bark of pine trees. Rich in antioxidants, they strengthen blood vessels. According to some tests, OPC's are fifty times as powerful as vitamin E.

Vitamin C— A powerful antioxidant that blocks the destructive activity of damaging free radicals. It helps regulate high blood pressure and LDL/HDL cholesterol levels. Vitamin C has been shown to help prevent atherosclerosis. Vitamin C-rich foods include cabbage, sweet peppers, strawberries, oranges, broccoli, tomatoes, guavas, currants, cantaloupe, and dark and leafy-green vegetables.

Vitamin D— New research, including studies from the University of Michigan Medical School, are now recognizing vitamin D as playing a role in the heart's pumping ability and cell structure. Foods with concentrated amounts of vitamin D are salmon, sardines, shrimp, milk, cod, and eggs. Vegetarian sources include Vitamin D-fortified cereals, soy milk, rice milk, and other non-dairy milks.

Vitamin E— Strengthens the heart muscle and keeps red blood cells from clumping. It works as an antioxidant. Links have been established between the increase of heart disease and a lack of vitamin E, a nutrient almost completely stripped from the American diet due to food processing. Food sources include filberts, almonds, wheat germ, sesame oil, sunflower oil, olive oil, peanuts, and sunflower seeds.

GET HEALTHY, AMERICA!

HEART-BUILDING FRESH JUICE

Magnesium Miracle Drink
　　1 stalk broccoli
　　1 carrot
　　1 handful each of kale and romaine
　　1 stalk of celery

• Push through a juicer and drink immediately.

6 The Lymphatic System

A healthy lymphatic system is an important component of optimum health. This system includes the bone marrow, lymph nodes, the spleen, and the thymus gland. Lymph fluid circulates throughout this system, constantly cleansing at the cellular level and carrying away waste products, toxins, and other debris.

Unlike blood, the lymphatic system doesn't have a heart to pump it through the body but rather relies on muscle movement. Walking is thought by many experts to be the best activity, but any movement you do will help "milk" the system and get lymph moving through the lymphatic vessels.

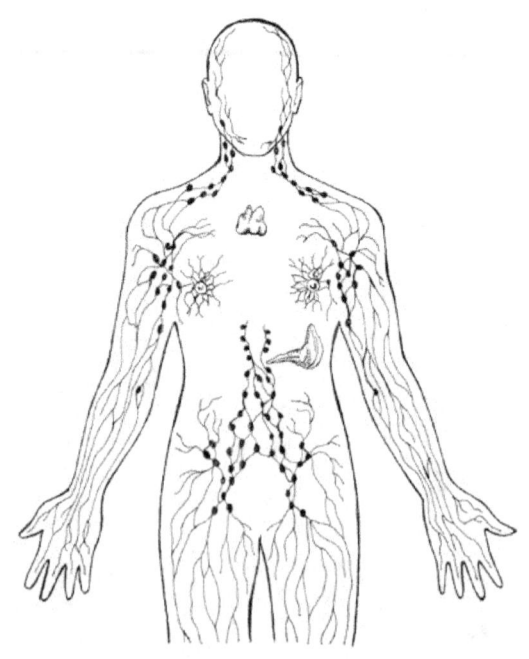

REBOUNDING & DRY-SKIN BRUSHING

Rebounding—jumping up and down on a small trampoline—is good for the lymphatic system because of the up-and-down movement that forces lymphatic fluid to move. The Journal of Cardiopulmonary Rehabilitation states, "The mini trampoline [rebounder] provides a convenient form of exercise with a major advantage being its apparent low level of trauma to the musculoskeletal system."[49]

Dry-skin brushing with movements toward the heart is good for freeing up stagnant lymph fluid. Some massage therapists specialize in manual lymph drainage massage, and this is a wonderful technique for lymph cleansing. See skin section in book for more information on dry-skin brushing.

ELIZABETH BAKER'S STORY ON REBOUNDING

"Elton Would Sit Me Down and Bounce Up and Down"

"When I was extremely sick back in the early 1980s, I was bedridden most of the time and moving very little. My dear husband, Elton, would have me sit on the rebounder. Then he would stand on it and put a leg on each side of me. Holding on, he would gently bounce up and down. My body would follow the motion. It was a great way to get my lymph flowing without my having to expend much energy."

WALK TO GET THE LYMPH MOVING

Get moving! Maybe you have heard the guidelines from health experts about walking 10,000 steps per day. It takes 2,000 steps to walk one mile, so 10,000 steps is close to five miles. If you are sedentary—from the car, to the office, to the computer, back to the car, and home to the TV—you may be averaging only 1,000 to 3,000 steps a day.

Dr. Joan Vernikos, former director of Life Sciences at NASA and astronaut trainer, discovered that when astronauts are in space, they age remarkably faster than when on earth. She has demonstrated that the gravity-free environment of space, contrary to that of our ancestors who were always walking, plowing and moving against gravity, causes unhealthy changes in the body. In her book, Sitting Kills Moving Heals, she explains that the current practice of sitting in cars and behind computers is extremely unhealthy and leads to disease.

NUTRITION FOR YOUR INTERNAL ORGANS

7 The Adrenal Glands

When you think about the adrenal glands, you should think about stress because many of the stress hormones are produced here. Whether it's the stress of taking an examination, being late to pick up the kids at daycare, recovering from illness, running from a chasing dog, or simply maintaining good energy everyday, the adrenal glands are involved.

The adrenals are a pair of triangular-shaped organs that are located above the kidneys. Reduced function of these important glands can result in depression, weakness, lethargy, dizziness, memory problems, and blood-sugar disorders. A diet low in sugar, alcohol, tobacco, and caffeine, and rich in whole grains, legumes, brown rice, cold-water fish, and raw fruits and vegetables is one of the best ways to nourish your adrenal glands. This kind of a diet will also give you the vitamins and minerals you need to deal with the stresses of daily living.

Kathleen didn't know at first why she was so fatigued and depressed. It turned out to be her adrenals.

—

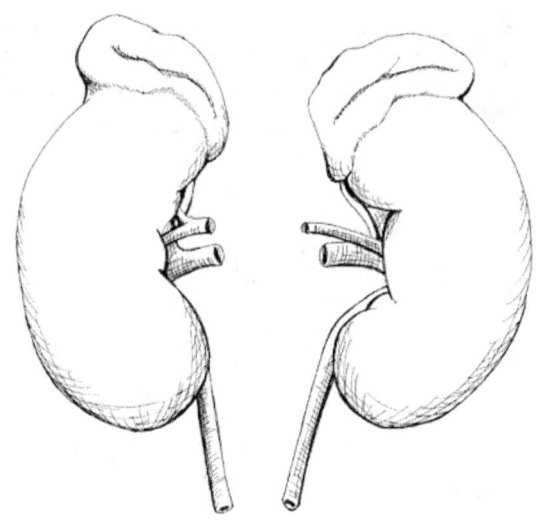

KATHLEEN'S STORY

"WHY WOULD ANYONE STAND UP WHEN THEY COULD SIT DOWN?"

Kathleen, a registered nurse at the Tahoma Clinic, worked closely with Dr. Wright. Her job was very demanding; dozens of clients passed through the clinic every day seeking her expertise. As she said, "It's important that I stay on top of my game since clients are counting on me." She was required to administer shots, start IVs, and generally be available to answer any questions that might arise regarding treatment plans.

She told me once, "I would watch the head nurse, Sandy, stand at the nursing station and talk on the phone. I couldn't help but stare at her and wonder why she was standing when she could sit in the chair beside her. For that matter, I wondered why anyone would sit down when they could lie down."

Kathleen was always a hard worker and told me that all the jobs she had ever had required that she perform "at her best," regardless of how she was feeling. But late in that year, she began feeling really strange. She said she was fuzzy headed, dizzy a lot, confused, and spaced out. Sometimes her words wouldn't come out right; she would jokingly say, "I put my tongue in backwards this morning!" or, "I just washed my mouth out, and I can't do a thing with it!" All joking aside, she was really not feeling well.

"Sometimes when I am sitting at the nursing station, I hold on to my chair because I feel like I could fall off! One night when I was cooking dinner, I had to lie down right in the middle of the kitchen floor for a couple of minutes. My son looked at me in shock and said, 'Mom, what's wrong with you?' I told him to just give me a couple minutes, and then I'd finish dinner."

She described the way she felt. "It's like I'm only half plugged in. Like a lamp that doesn't have a complete connection. If someone would just push the plug in all the way, I think the circuit would be completed, and I'd get the energy I need."

So Kathleen scheduled a brief appointment with Dr. Wright (yes, staff had to schedule, too). Among other things, he ordered an adrenal test, which showed that she had *hypoadrenalism*—adrenal fatigue. Since these glands are important for energy, it was no wonder Kathleen was feeling poorly.

Dr. Wright put Kathleen on a program that included natural adrenal supplementation, a diet rich in adrenal-supporting nutrients, and other specific supplements.

Kathleen also began juicing three times a day as a New Year's resolution. She juiced mostly leafy greens and produce rich in the B vitamin pantothenic acid and vitamin C. And she stuck with the juicing faithfully. Within three months, all of her symptoms of fatigue had totally disappeared. She attributed much of her renewed health to her stringent juicing program. She was feeling her normal self again, and since that time, she has always shared her personal story with anyone suffering with low energy and fatigue.

ACTION PLAN FOR HEALTHY ADRENAL GLANDS
GENERAL RECOMMENDATIONS

• Oftentimes, people with weak adrenals become dizzy when they squat down, then stand up suddenly. Here is a simple home test that can help you determine the health of your adrenals:

Normally, systolic blood pressure (the first number in the measurement of blood pressure—120/80) is approximately 10 points higher when you are standing than when you are lying down. If the adrenal glands are not functioning properly, however, this may not be the case.

Take and compare two blood pressure readings—one while lying down and one while standing. First, lie down and rest for five minutes. Then take your blood pressure. Stand up and immediately take your blood pressure again. If your blood pressure reading is lower after you stand up, suspect reduced adrenal gland function. The degree to which the blood pressure drops upon standing is often proportionate to the degree of hypoadrenalism.[50]

DIETARY TIPS

• Caffeine-containing beverages stress the adrenal glands. Try replacing coffee with a coffee substitute (found in health food stores and made from various grains) or herbal tea (dandelion tea is a tasty coffee substitute).

- Replace caffeine-containing soft drinks with pure water or other natural beverages.

- Stop eating sugar—a known vitamin B robber.

BENEFICIAL VITAMINS, MINERALS, AND HERBS

Chinese Ginseng and **Siberian Ginseng**— Tonics that balance the body's response to acute and chronic stress, you'll find ginseng in capsules, tinctures, and teas. For guaranteed potency, look for standardized ginseng. Standardized is a term that means a substance contains a guaranteed amount of a certain botanical constituent.

Other Immune-Supporting Herbs—Echinacea, Pau d'Arco, Hyssop, and Mullein, all available in supplemental forms.

Pantothenic Acid— This adrenal-specific anti-stress B vitamin is stored in high amounts in the adrenal glands and is needed for their proper function. Food sources of pantothenic acid include beef, brewer's yeast, molasses, eggs, legumes, mushrooms, nuts, royal jelly, avocado, filberts, broccoli, and whole-wheat.

Vitamin B Complex— The entire vitamin B family is important for proper adrenal function. High-potency vitamin B capsules will contain the correct amounts of the major B vitamins. Your diet should contain vitamin B-rich foods: wheat germ, whole-grain breads and cereals, nuts, seeds, dark and leafy-green vegetables, most fruits, and vegetables.

Vitamin C—This vitamin is critical for proper adrenal function, aiding in the production of anti-stress hormones. Daily supplementation, in addition to a good diet, may be beneficial. Foods are peppers, oranges, cantaloupe, and strawberries.

Zinc— This mineral boosts immune function. Zinc-rich foods include oysters, turkey, pumpkin, and whole-grain cereals.

GET HEALTHY, AMERICA!

ADRENAL GLAND FRESH JUICE

Green Energy Booster
One stalk broccoli
One handful of mixed greens
One bunch parsley
You may add an apple or a slice of ginger for flavor.

- Push through juicer and drink immediately.

8 The Gallbladder

The *gallbladder* is a pear-shaped pouch located just under the liver. It holds bile that squirts into the intestines to aid digestion. Gallbladder disease (*gallstones*) develops when abnormal concentrations of bile from the liver form hard stones that can become lodged in the *bile ducts*. As many as twenty million Americans have gallstones.[51]

Eating fried or fatty foods can aggravate the gallbladder and cause pain and vomiting. Symptoms also include severe pain in the abdomen which shoots into the back and shoulder area. Common medical treatment is removal of the gallbladder.

Gallstones are often a result of food allergy. James C. Breneman, M.D., past chairman of the Food Allergy Committee of the American College of Allergists, reported, "Gallbladder attacks could be completely avoided by eliminating allergenic foods from the diet."[52] Common offending foods are eggs, wheat, milk, oranges and peanuts.

Another review of scientific literature relates food to gallbladder disease. In one study, it was found that "consumption of carbohydrates in refined form increases bile cholesterol saturation. The risk of gallstones might be reduced by avoidance of refined carbohydrate foods."[53]

ACTION PLAN FOR A HEALTHY GALLBLADDER
GENERAL RECOMMENDATIONS

- A gallbladder flush can be helpful to clear this organ. Following is one version of a gallbladder flush from *Gut Solutions* by Brenda Watson, ND:

Caution—Please use caution and physician direction for the below flush, which can be done two to three times yearly.

Monday through Friday–Drink as much organic apple juice as possible. Eat normally. Continue to take your usual medications and/or supplements.

Saturday–Eat your lunch as usual. At about 3 p.m., drink one tablespoon Epsom salts in ¼ cup warm water. Follow this with freshly squeezed grapefruit or orange juice to help improve elimination. At 5 p.m., repeat the process—Epson salts and grapefruit or orange juice afterward, if desired. For dinner, eat citrus fruit or juices (freshly squeezed). Before bed, drink ½ cup cold-pressed extra virgin olive oil mixed with ½ cup lemon juice. In bed, lie on your right side, with knees pulled close to your chest, for half an hour.

Sunday Morning–Upon rising (an hour before breakfast), take one tablespoon Epsom salts in warm water. This will help flush material out of the liver/gallbladder into the intestinal tract.[54]

You will find more versions of this flush on the internet or in nutritional cleansing books.

DIETARY TIPS

- Alfalfa, dandelion, horsetail, and ginger root (in tea or capsules) all help cleanse the liver and gallbladder.

- Consume apples, which contain pectin and aid digestion.

- Eliminate drinks and foods containing white sugar.

- Increase vegetable consumption, including vegetables with their skins.

- Many large scale studies have shown that people who eat the highest intake of vegetables are significantly less likely to have gallstone symptoms compared to those who eat few vegetables.

- Lemon juice, beet juice, shredded beets, and pears are all cleansing to the gallbladder.

- Reduce saturated fat and meat intake.

- Replace all white-flour products with whole grains.

BENEFICIAL VITAMINS, MINERALS, AND HERBS

Choline and **Inositol**— (Members of the B vitamin family) help with cholesterol metabolism and liver/gallbladder function. They are available in supplemental form. Choline is present in eggs, beef, and navy beans. Inositol is in nuts, beans, and whole wheat.

Lecithin— Granules emulsify fat and aid digestion. Available in natural food stores in packages, it can be added to smoothies.

Multi-enzyme— Capsules help digest food. See healthtreasurechest.com under the products and supplements section for a line of enzymes.

Peppermint oil— Helps to cleanse the gallbladder. Available in liquids and tinctures in natural food stores.

GET HEALTHY, AMERICA!

GALLBLADDER FRESH JUICE

Cleansing Juice Cocktail
　　1 small lemon, peeled
　　1 slice of fresh ginger (size of a quarter)
　　1 apple
　　½ small beet

- Push through a juicer and drink immediately.

9 The Kidneys and Urinary System

The kidneys, each about the size of a fist, are located at the lowest level of the rib cage on both sides of the body. Their major function is to remove waste products and excess fluid from the body via the urine. This process helps maintain a stable balance of body chemicals. The health of the kidneys and urinary tract is directly affected by what we eat and drink.

> "Kidney stones are abnormal accumulations of mineral salts which form in the kidney but may lodge anywhere in the urinary tract. They can be the size of sand or gravel or as large as bird eggs. Often removed surgically, they can reappear if the diet is not improved."[55]

Bladder infections are usually caused when *E. coli bacteria*, a normal inhabitant in the colon, invades the sterile urinary tract. This bacterium attaches itself to the bladder lining and digs in, resulting in pain and/or urinary frequency. Common treatment with antibiotics can set the stage for repeat bacterial infections, perhaps involving bacteria other than E. coli. Symptoms include urge to "go," burning, and painful urination.

ACTION PLAN FOR HEALTHY KIDNEYS
GENERAL RECOMMENDATIONS

- Drink the number of ounces equal to ½ your body weight in fresh, filtered water every day to keep the kidneys and bladder working properly. For instance, if you weigh 150 pounds, you would drink seventy-five ounces of water daily.

DIETARY TIPS

- Cranberries acidify the urine, destroying bacteria. The fruits or juice are good for bladder infections. Only buy sugar-free cranberry juice.

- Fresh celery and parsley act as natural diuretics, stimulating urination. Eat them fresh, or add them to fresh vegetable juices.

- Lemon is a known kidney/bladder cleanser. Add to purified water.

BENEFICIAL VITAMINS, MINERALS, AND HERBS

D-Mannose—A simple sugar occurring naturally in some plants, it is rapidly excreted in the urine. D-mannose adheres to bacteria in the bladder, preventing them from sticking to the lining. Bacteria can then be expelled in the urine. D-mannose does not interfere with blood sugar regulation.

Other Beneficial Herbs—Taken as teas or capsules, include parsley, watermelon seed, marshmallow root, and nettle.

Uva Ursi— This herb has been used for centuries, and Native Americans used it as a remedy for urinary tract infections.

GET HEALTHY, AMERICA!

KIDNEY CLEANSING FRESH JUICE

Green Mania Kidney Builder
2 stalks celery
1 handful parsley
½ cucumber

- Put through a juicer and drink immediately.

1 0 The Liver

Here is a bit of nostalgia for baby boomers. Do you remember "Carter's Little Liver Pills"? I do. Their TV ads were sandwiched somewhere between "Superman" and "What's My Line?" A recent article in *Time* Magazine read,

> One of the most familiar of all trade names was booked for a major operation last week. The Federal Trade Commission told the manufacturers of Carter's Little Liver Pills to cut the word 'liver' out of the product name ...
>
> ···Carter sought his raw materials in nature. Podophyllum resin, or podophyllin, is the resin of the dried root of the mandrake or May apple; Carter combined this with the dried juice of aloes. He chose as his trademark an overstuffed black crow, which gave a nice zoological balance to Bull Durham's bull on the nation's barns ...
>
> ···Half a century later, a new advertising technique gave the sexagenarian business an added boost. The ominous crow was retired; the slogan became "Wake up your liver bile!" Jingles urged readers and radio listeners: "When you feel sour and sunk, and the world looks punk ... Take a Carter's Little Liver Pill." Carter's went on to claim that the increased liver bile would enable the pill-taker to overeat and overindulge in "good times" without morning-after regrets, to wake up "clear-eyed and steady-nerved," "feeling just wonderful, and "alert and ready for work."
>
> ···Its ruling last week not only forbade Carter products to use the word "liver" in the name of its pills, but told Carter's to stop claiming that its pills are specific remedies for conditions in which

an individual feels "down-and-out, blue, down-in-the-dumps, worn out, sunk, logy, depressed, sluggish, allin, listless, mean, low, cross, tired, stuffy, heavy, miserable, sour, grouchy, irritable, cranky, peevish, fagged out, dull, sullen, what's-the-use, bogged down, grumpy, run down or gloomy."

···The FTC left one door open. Carter's can still recommend its pills for such miseries to the extent that any of them can be temporarily relieved by an evacuation of the bowels. [56]

The liver is certainly a major organ of detoxification, and it looks like in 1868, Dr. Samuel Carter of Erie, PA., knew it! Whether or not his aloe and mandrake pills had any action on the liver can be debated (although aloe and mandrake are listed in many herbal references books as helpful to the liver), but one thing is for sure—a healthy liver is central to good health!

THE WORK OF THE LIVER

Because of the liver's ability to detoxify the body, many natural health clinics worldwide use therapies to cleanse and support this organ. However, there would be less need for liver support and cleansing if the diet was high in organic, whole, and unprocessed foods. This type of diet takes the excessive load off the liver by decreasing the amount of toxins entering the body. The liver is the only organ that can regenerate itself if it is damaged.[57]

ACTION PLAN FOR A HEALTHY LIVER
GENERAL RECOMMENDATIONS

- Food choices are very important for a healthy liver. Because the liver is the organ that does the majority of body detoxification, eating a natural diet free of preservatives, additives, and chemical-laden foods is important.

DIETARY TIPS

- Choose a whole-food, organic diet rich in fiber.

- No alcohol. Cirrhosis of the liver, a serious disease involving scarring, can be caused by excessive alcohol consumption.

BENEFICIAL VITAMINS, MINERALS, AND HERBS

Choline— (From the B vitamin family) is helpful for a fatty liver. Food sources include egg yolks, lecithin, soybeans, and whole-grains. Granulated lecithin which has choline is available in natural food stores.

Freshly prepared juices—Should include beets, lemons, and papaya.

Herbal cleansing kits— For liver detoxification are available in natural food stores or at healthtreasurechest.com. These are generally very effective. Follow instructions in kit, which should also include dietary recommendations.

Milk thistle herb— Is commonly used to help the liver regenerate and to protect it from damage. Available in natural food stores.

GET HEALTHY, AMERICA!

LIVER-BUILDING FRESH JUICE

Love Your Liver Elixir
1 medium beet
½ lemon
1 handful parsley
1 small apple

- Put all through a juicer and drink immediately.

11 The Pancreas, Spleen, Thymus, and Thyroid

THE PANCREAS

The pancreas is discussed extensively in the Hypoglycemia/Diabetes section.

THE SPLEEN

The spleen is the largest mass of lymphatic tissue in the body and is an important part of the immune system. It filters blood, removing old red blood cells that need replacing. People who have had their spleen removed tend to be more prone to illness because of the role this organ plays in immunity.

For a healthy spleen, follow a natural diet, emphasizing immune-building principles—whole, unprocessed foods with plenty of fruits and vegetables.

Beneficial foods and herbs for the spleen are carrots, beets, cucumbers, parsley, cabbage, potatoes, onions, and dandelion.

THE THYMUS

The thymus gland is located below the neck in the center of the body about two finger-widths below the notch where the right and left clavicles meet. "The thymus is the site where T cells mature. T cells play a role in immunity by secreting interleukin-1, interleukin-2, and interferon, as well as activating B cells so that they produce antibodies."[58]

Since the thymus is part of the immune system, it is critical to assess anything that may be compromising it. A poor diet and stress are considered to be major factors that suppress immunity. Vitamin E, selenium, and beta-carotene can help protect the thymus. Beneficial herbs such as echinacea root, goldenseal, and myrrh help increase the activity of the white blood cells.

Good food choices for the thymus and immune system are pumpkin seeds, citrus fruits, carrots, raw nuts and seeds, oatmeal, chicken, and garbanzo beans.

THE THYROID

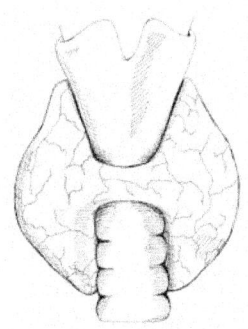

Hypothyroidism, or an underproduction of thyroid hormone, is a common condition of the thyroid gland. Symptoms include slow heartbeat, muscle weakness, fatigue, dry and/or yellow skin, inability to tolerate cold, and weight gain. *Hyperthyroidism* is a condition where the body produces too much thyroid hormone. It is not as common as hypothyroidism.

The function of the thyroid gland is to take iodine, found in many foods, and convert it into the thyroid hormones: thyroxine (T_4) and triiodothyronine (T_3). Thyroid cells are the only cells in the body which can absorb iodine.

These cells combine iodine and the amino acid tyrosine to make T_3 and T_4. T_3 and T_4 are then released into the blood stream and are transported throughout the body where they control metabolism (conversion of oxygen and calories to energy). Every cell in the body depends upon thyroid hormones for regulation of their metabolism. The normal thyroid gland produces about 80% T_4 and about 20% T3, however, T3 possesses about four times the hormone "strength" as T4.[59]

ACTION PLAN FOR A HEALTHY THYROID
GENERAL RECOMMENDATIONS

- Taking your underarm body temperature will give you an idea of your thyroid health. Shake down a thermometer to 96° before going to bed. In the morning as soon as you wake up, put the thermometer under your arm and remain in bed for 10 minutes. Normal underarm temperatures average 97.8° to 98.2°. Anything below that could indicate thyroid insufficiency.

DIETARY TIPS

- Follow a whole-food diet, low in sugar and devoid of refined, junk foods. Follow a moderate exercise program and drink only pure water.

BENEFICIAL VITAMINS, MINERALS, AND HERBS

B-vitamins— Are needed by the thyroid. Dark, leafy green vegetables are a good source.

Iodine— Is necessary for a healthy thyroid and is present in seafood, iodized salt, seaweed (kelp), and mustard greens.

Tyrosine— An amino acid, is critical for the thyroid. Sources include carob, bean sprouts, soybeans, peanuts, oats, watercress, chives, pumpkin seeds, and cabbage.

Vitamins A, E, and **C**— Stimulate thyroid production. Foods rich in these vitamins are papaya and bell peppers (C); sunflower seeds, almonds, and olives (E); and carrots, liver, and spinach (A).

Zinc— Aids in thyroid production. Foods rich in zinc are pumpkin seeds, beef, lamb, yogurt, and peas.

GET HEALTHY, AMERICA!

THYROID FRESH JUICE

Thyroid Energizer
One handful each of cabbage, spinach, and romaine lettuce
Small bunch of chives
2 carrots
½ an apple

- Push through a juicer and drink immediately.

NUTRITION FOR NATURAL BEAUTY

1 2 The Eyes

The eyes—two of the most complex organs of the body—require good nutrition to function properly. A major contributor to eye problems is a poor diet full of dead, preserved, and stripped foods. Making sure to feed your eyes properly today could save you serious eye problems as you age.

SUNLIGHT & EYES

John Ott, PhD, began taking time lapse pictures of plants under fluorescent lights in his basement in 1927. He found that plants thrived, or withered and died, depending on the type of light they received.

Ott turned his attention towards studying the beneficial effects of full-spectrum lighting. Sunlight is considered full spectrum; in moderation, sunlight improves immunity, prevents disease, increases intelligence, stimulates our metabolism, and boosts energy levels.

Full spectrum of the sun's light rays has been shown to reduce the risk of getting sick and lowers blood pressure, among other benefits. The problem is that getting adequate sunlight isn't easy these days. Most of us suffer from sunlight starvation. Dr. Ott advocated the continual need for sunlight in our lives and to replace standard lighting with a better full spectrum sunlight variety. [60]

As a society, we are living indoors and under synthetic light more and more. Many people get almost no natural light. We are conditioned to always wear sunglasses. A few lighting manufacturers have built indoor lights that approximate natural daylight in intensity and color spectrum. These lights are called *full-spectrum lights* and are very useful in light therapy for SAD (Seasonal Affective Disorder).

In keeping with Dr. Ott's findings, many health care practitioners believe and teach that a moderate amount of sunlight on the body and into the eyes is not only healthy, but necessary (in moderation; a few minutes in the morning and/or late afternoon when the harmful rays are being filtered by the earth's atmosphere).

MACULAR DEGENERATION

According to the National Eye Institutes, *macular degeneration* is the leading cause of vision loss and blindness in Americans aged 65 and older. "It is a disease of the central part of the eye, and characterized by accumulation of oxidized fat (*lipofuscin*) and thinning of the macular pigment."[61]

Macular degeneration is usually a slow process that sometimes can appear suddenly. This painless loss of vision begins from the middle of the cornea, so sight is reduced in the center of the vision area. Early signs of vision loss can include seeing shadowy areas in your central vision or experiencing unusually fuzzy or distorted vision.[62] There is a definite connection between nutrition and the prevention of macular degeneration. In one study, both macular disease and blindness were reduced in those with intermediate damage by taking vitamin C, beta -carotene, vitamin E, and zinc on a daily basis.

Additionally, some studies have found that people who had the lowest serum levels of *lycopene,* a carotenoid, are significantly more likely to have macular degeneration when compared to those with the highest levels. Tomatoes are a good source of lycopene, and several new studies suggest that they may help protect the eyes by preventing macular degeneration. Dark greens (such as spinach) are also important. Why not give up nutrient-deficient iceberg lettuce in your salads in favor of health-promoting spinach?

GLAUCOMA

Glaucoma is a group of eye diseases that gradually steal sight without warning. In the early stages of the disease, there may be no symptoms. Experts estimate that half of the people affected by glaucoma may not know they have it.[63]

While some say that glaucoma is genetic, it actually can be the result of nutritional deficiencies. The eyes are one of the first areas of the body that are affected by a lack of nutrition because they are so sensitive.

ELIZABETH BAKER'S EYE EXERCISES

"I'VE DONE THESE EXERCISES FOR OVER TWO DECADES NOW"

As recorded at a Get Healthy, America! Seminar, 1-7-07
"I've done these exercises for over two decades now. They have helped me keep my eyes strong and my vision clear. Maybe they will help you.

Stretch your right arm straight out in front of you. Keep your head stationary at all times, looking straight forward. Only move your eyes. With both eyes, stare at the tip of your index finger. Slowly bring your finger toward your nose. Touch your nose with your finger, keeping both eyes focused on the finger the entire time. Slowly straighten your arm after a few seconds to the starting position, arm straight out in front of you. Repeat this several times.

Next, bring extended arm/index finger to the 2 o'clock position, and repeat the exercise. Keep head straight forward. Finally, bring the index finger to the 5 o'clock position, and repeat. Do this also with the extended left arm/finger, bringing the finger to the 7 o'clock and 10 o'clock positions."

———

Eye exercises such as those mentioned above can benefit your brain in addition to benefiting your eyes. Researchers from Manchester Metropolitan University in England report that after hearing a list of words, those who moved their eyes side-to-side for thirty seconds correctly remembered more than ten percent more words and falsely recognized about fifteen percent fewer "lure" words, compared to those who moved their eyes up-and-down or did nothing.

Why would moving your eyes influence your memory? The researchers suspect it's because the horizontal eye movements cause the two hemispheres of the brain to interact more, and communication between the left and right brain hemispheres is known to help us remember certain things.

The researchers aren't sure whether the eye movements will help people in their daily lives …but it's certainly worth a try the next time you've misplaced your keys or forgotten your grocery list at home.[64]

ACTION PLAN FOR HEALTHY EYES
GENERAL RECOMMENDATIONS

- Research suggests that antioxidants reduce your risk of developing eye diseases. Specific antioxidants can be of particular benefit.

Eat a well-balanced diet with plenty of whole, raw, unprocessed fruits, vegetables, seeds, herbs, and spices.

DIETARY TIPS

- Every day, eat foods rich in the phytochemicals *lutein* and *zeaxanthin:* dark, leafy-green and deep yellow vegetables from land and sea, blueberries, and corn.

- Make vitamin A foods a regular part of your diet. These include carrots, yams, sweet potatoes, apricots, pumpkin, papaya, broccoli, spinach, kale, collard greens, yellow squash, and beet greens.

BENEFICIAL VITAMINS, MINERALS, AND HERBS

Eyebright— When used as an eyewash or compress or in conjunction with capsules, this herb strengthens the eye.

Ginkgo Biloba— An herb known to improve capillary circulation in the eyes. Available in natural food stores, it is found in capsules, teas, and tinctures.

Lutein— The macular region of the retina is composed of two dietary components, lutein and zeaxanthin. According to researchers the macular pigment protects the photoreceptor cells from light damage by absorbing blue light. The macular pigment can be increased by improving the intake of foods that are rich in lutein and zeaxanthin or by supplementation.[65]

Red Raspberry Tea— Tea made from raspberry leaves. Use four tea bags to make a strong tea and moisten a cloth with it; place over eyes for redness/irritation. This tea is available at most natural food stores.

Taurine— An amino acid present in protein that works in conjunction with zinc in maintaining eye function. It is present in the retina of the eye in high concentrations. Taurine rich foods include eggs, fish oils, and milk.

Vitamin A— Protects the eye from free-radical damage. Even a slight deficiency can cause tired eyes, sensitivity to light, dry eyelids, susceptibility to infections, possible ulcerations, and irreversible blindness in extreme cases. To avoid the above symptoms, consume carotenoid-rich foods: spinach, kale, broccoli, cauliflower, cabbage, mustard greens, collard greens, carrots, cantaloupe, pumpkin, and yellow squash.

Vitamin B Complex— A lack of the B vitamins can cause itching, burning, light sensitivity and bloodshot, watering eyes. B-2 deficiency can result in color disturbance, inability to see part of an image or printed page, halos around lights or objects, and spots floating in front of the eyes. Foods rich in the family of B vitamins include whole cereal grains, dark and leafy greens, raw fruits, and brewer's yeast.

Vitamin C— This vitamin is concentrated in the eyes. In the Nutrition and Vision Project, a subsidy of the federally funded Nurses' Health Study, it was found that those who used vitamin C supplements for 10 or more years were 64% less likely to have cloudy lenses than those who never used vitamin C.[66]

Vitamin E— Vitamin E is a good antioxidant that is eye-protective. Sources include sunflower seeds, hazelnuts, peanuts, almonds, and mangos.

GET HEALTHY, AMERICA!

SEE-CLEARLY JUICE

Carrot Cocktail
2 carrots
1 handful spinach
1 handful kale
1 handful collard greens

- Push through juicer and drink immediately.

1 3 The Skin

Your skin is actually an organ—the largest one in your body. The skin helps maintain correct body temperature; protects all your internal organs from external influences; and helps you to perceive stimuli such as hot/cold, rough/smooth, and hard/soft. Skin is important for the manufacturing of vitamin D, which occurs when the rays of the sun make contact with the skin.

As a natural consequence of aging, the skin begins to lose its elasticity, and wrinkles form over time. While some amount of wrinkling is normal due to age and genetics, it is possible to slow down the extent and rate at which that wrinkling will occur.

Loretta has certainly figured out a way to keep her skin looking beautiful. I met her on my most recent visit to the Optimum Health Institute in San Diego in 2007.

LORETTA—A MOVIE STAR'S STORY

"MY SECRET? I EXERCISE MY FACE!"

Loretta was once a movie star. She had a youthful face, gorgeous skin, and a tight chin. I was amazed that she was almost seventy years old. She looked about fifty!

Many of the middle-aged guests at the facility were very concerned about their sagging faces, so we asked her to tell us her secret. She was happy to oblige.

"You've got to exercise your face!"

She told us to hang our heads slightly over the edge of a bed (protecting our necks) and then do "chin-ups."

"You gently drop your head backwards, then raise it up a few inches, all the while focusing on the muscles in the chin and neck. I do thirty to forty chin-ups several days a week."

———

Loretta explained why facial exercises work. Curious about her comment, I did some research and found the following:

> Facial muscles elongate just like the muscles in the arms, thighs and buttocks. As a result of gravity and atrophy, muscles in the face will have elongated about one-half inch by the time most people have reached the age of 55. Even though we talk, sing or laugh, the muscles continue to soften and become lax; it's only when the facial muscles are specifically exercised that they begin to plump up and support your skin better, responding in the face similarly to other muscles in the body.[67]

If you have back or neck problems, consult with your healthcare practitioner before doing these exercises.

DRY-SKIN BRUSHING FOR REJUVENATION

The skin replenishes itself continually. Large amounts of body waste are eliminated through the skin daily. If the blood is full of toxins, that toxicity can manifest as a poor complexion, skin eruptions, and a generally unhealthy appearance.

Dry skin brushing is a technique that helps the skin eliminate toxins. Use a natural bristle brush with a long handle. Brush when your skin is dry, before taking a shower or bath. Begin by brushing only one or two minutes a day. Gradually build up to several minutes daily.

Begin by brushing in long, sweeping strokes from the feet upward and from the hands toward the shoulders and on the torso in an upward direction. Always brush toward the heart. Avoid areas where there are skin problems or sensitive areas.

HERE ARE SOME BENEFITS OF DRY-SKIN BRUSHING:

- It helps remove layers of old, dead skin.
- It increases blood circulation to the skin and underlying organs.
- The stimulation helps to eliminate toxic waste materials.
- It helps with muscle tone and more even distribution of fat deposits.
- Lymphatic circulation is increased.

DANDRUFF TIPS

Dandruff is a form of dry skin of the scalp. While TV advertising claims that dandruff-stopping shampoos can correct the problem, it usually starts on the inside. The best way to stop it is to change the diet to a more healthful, natural one.

A major cause of dandruff is a diet with too much hydrogenated fat and fried foods, too much sugar, and little or no healthy essential fatty acids. Replace processed foods with those that are high in essential fatty acids (EFAs) such as cold-pressed vegetable oils, olive oil, and fresh nuts and seeds.

Poor water intake also is usually an underlying issue. Food allergies and deficiencies of B vitamins, beta-carotene, and minerals such as zinc are all possible causes of dandruff. Many people with dandruff, like the mailman in the story below, have some serious food issues.

THE MAILMAN STORY

"I'LL TAKE THE BIG ONE"

Some years ago, I was in a convenience store to pay for gasoline. In front of me in line was a mailman who had stopped for lunch. He was carrying a couple of doughnuts and a candy bar. When they asked what size soda he would like, he said, "I'll take the big one."

I noticed that the shoulders of his blue work suit were covered with white, flaky dandruff…really bad dandruff! His face appeared very oily, and he had flaky skin in the corners of his nose. He didn't look very well. I had just begun my studies in nutrition and had read about natural help for dandruff.

Dandruff is generally linked to eating too much sugar, too many carbohydrates, and a deficiency of the B-vitamins and essential fatty acids.

Twenty-five years later, I still remember that mailman. I wish now that I had been bold enough to tell him that his food choices that day, if indicative of the way he ate habitually, were causing him to be nutrient deficient and were killing him. But then, hindsight is always better than foresight. And some folks don't appreciate the unsolicited advice of strangers, no matter how well-meaning!

NUTRITION FOR STRETCH MARKS

Stretch marks are wavy stripes that appear on the abdomen or other areas of the body as a result of rapid weight gain or pregnancy. Body builders often get stretch marks on their upper arms where they have built excessive muscle. Vitamin E is an excellent remedy for stretch marks.

Here is a natural formula that can be rubbed on stretch marks:

½ cup virgin olive oil
¼ cup liquid aloe vera
Liquid from four capsules vitamin E
Liquid from four capsules vitamin A

- Mix all ingredients and refrigerate. Once or more daily, rub on areas where you have stretch marks.

ELIZABETH BAKER'S FAVORITE FACIAL MOISTURIZER

"I've always said that oils are not the complete answer for facial treatments. Underneath the top layer of the skin there may still be dryness, even after applications of a rich, heavy oil. Since oil and water do not mix, you must have an agent that will blend the two. Food-grade glycerin is the key. The skin should be slightly acidic to kill any bacteria present and help stop minor infections from slight abrasions.

Here is the formula I have used for many years (a fraction of the cost of fancy, department store varieties):

One part glycerin
One part hydrogen peroxide (inexpensive, drugstore variety will do)
One part vinegar (preferably raw apple cider)
One part olive oil (I prefer olive oil because it is biblical, has been around for thousands of years, and experts still recommend it).

- Put the ingredients in a sterile bottle, shaking before use. Use sparingly, morning/night or as desired. You may add one-half part rosewater for a pleasant scent. Apricot oil also adds a lovely fragrance. These ingredients are all readily available in a drugstore or pharmacy."[68]

PAAVO AIROLA'S F-PLUS FORMULA

Paavo Airola, ND, PhD, famous Canadian naturopath and natural healer, developed the following formula for moisturizing the skin:

2 tbsp. sesame oil   2 tbsp. almond oil
1 tbsp. olive oil   2,000 IU vitamin E
2 tbsp. avocado oil   100,000 IU vitamin A

Pour all the oils into a sterile jar. Break open the vitamin E and Vitamin A capsules by puncturing them with a sterilized needle and squeeze the contents into the jar. Put the lid on tightly and shake well. Keep the oil mixture in the refrigerator for later use. Since vitamin A can smell fishy, a synthetic form can be used. [69]

OLD SCAR COMBINATION

While reviewing the healing powers of helichrysum (everlasting) for the herbal section of this book, I found this interesting formula:

1/8 teaspoon pure (essential) helichrysum oil
1/8 teaspoon pure sage oil
3 teaspoons pure rose hip seed oil
3 teaspoons pure hazelnut oil

Apply two to three times daily to old scars until you see results. While lotions, potions, oils, and facial formulas are very beneficial, you can also improve the appearance of your skin and face by changing old habits. Mentor Elizabeth Baker frequently talked about frowning and its negative effects. I never really thought about changing my own facial expressions until I'd heard her story.

ELIZABETH BAKER TALKS ABOUT WRINKLES

"Habits that we developed at a young age can stay with us for life. They simply become normal. Many years ago, a young friend of mine (in her late 50s, which seems young to me) would habitually wrinkle up her face into a frown when she was intense and wanted to get her point across.

When I called her attention to it, she graciously received my suggestions and began concentrating on not frowning. It has made a tremendous improvement in her appearance, and the wrinkles on her face are far less noticeable.

I say it is just as easy to look bright-eyed and to lift your brows when you talk. That way, you don't make wrinkles. I do eye exercises every day to keep the muscles around my eyes from sagging: squint your eyes together as tightly as you can, then open your eyes as wide as you can. Do this several times. Then concentrate on positive and pleasant thoughts and you can train your face to be in a smiling, rather than a frowning position."

ACTION PLAN FOR BEAUTIFUL, HEALTHY SKIN
GENERAL RECOMMENDATIONS

- Many factors determine the rate and extent to which our skin will age—nutrition, muscle tone, habitual facial expressions, choices of skin care products, and amount of exposure to the sun. Heredity also has an influence. While you can't change your genetics, you can make lifestyle changes to keep your skin looking healthy.

- Be sure to drink enough water. Divide your body weight in half and drink that many ounces of filtered water every day. If you experience thirst, you are already dehydrated. Drink a few ounces of purified water every twenty minutes throughout the day. Also avoid use of alcoholic beverages and caffeinated beverages because they dry out the skin.

DIETARY TIPS

- Almonds— Almonds are rich in vitamin E, which has antioxidants that protect against skin damage and premature aging of facial tissue.

- Avocado— This creamy food is rich in essential oils and B-complex vitamins. Mashed avocado can be rubbed on the face and left for twenty minutes.

- Flaxseed Oil— Rich in the omega-3s, flaxseed and flaxseed oils hydrate the skin.

- Mangos— Mangos are very rich in vitamin A, which is good for prematurely aging skin.

- Wheatgerm— Wheat germ is a good source of biotin, a B vitamin that is crucial to skin health. Sprinkle wheat germ on yogurt, salads, casseroles or your other favorite foods for a tasty way to get more biotin in your diet.

BENEFICIAL VITAMINS, MINERALS, AND HERBS

Cod Liver Oil— Cod liver oil is known to erase wrinkles. Ingest ½ to 1 tablespoon a day, plain or mixed in a little yogurt, with a pinch of sea salt for palatability.

Herbs— Excellent in forms such as rubs, wraps, oils, or in emollients. Alfalfa (a natural cleanser and ingredient in many face masks and lotions), chamomile (reduces appearance of wrinkles), horsetail (used topically for skin conditions), red raspberry (rich in minerals and vitamins that promote the health of the skin), and thyme (nourishes skin).

MSM (Methylsulfonylmethane)— A naturally occurring sulfur compound found in our bodies as well as in many common beverages and foods. It is a natural wrinkle reducer. If you have a sulfur allergy, do not use MSM without your doctor's permission.

Protection— While a small amount of sun on the skin is healthy, protect your face from too much sun exposure with a natural sunscreen that can be found at most natural food stores. Even with the sunscreen on, try to keep the sun off your face with a hat.

Vitamin A— Needed for healthy skin, vitamin A is used in the treatment of acne by many practitioners.

Vitamin C— Important in healing wounds of the skin. Vitamin C is used in expensive cosmetics because it rejuvenates the skin and makes it appear younger by working as an antioxidant.

Vitamin D— Formed in the body in part by interaction with sunlight and may play a role in skin pigmentation. Applying this vitamin topically can have a positive effect on skin health since it is well absorbed.

Essential Fatty Acids— Help smooth rough skin and prevent free-radical damage. A pharmaceutical grade (no mercury) EFA capsule is available through healthtreasurechest.com. Go to products and supplements.

GET HEALTHY, AMERICA!

HEALTHY SKIN JUICE

Best Beauty Drink
    1 carrot
    1 handful parsley
    Slice of ginger ¼ inch wide
    ¼ a lemon without peel

- Push through a juicer and drink immediately.

① ④ The Hair

Your hair requires good nutrition in order to be shiny and strong. Make sure you are eating plenty of fruits and vegetables of bright color because they are rich in *flavonoids*—powerful antioxidants that plants produce to protect themselves from parasites, bacteria, and cell injury. Fruits and vegetables are rich in antioxidants that provide protection and nutrition to the follicles of the hair.

To encourage blood circulation to the scalp, brush your hair daily with a natural bristle brush. You can also lie on a slant board for several minutes daily. A slant board is an adjustable board with a mechanism to raise your feet higher than your head. During your session, massage your scalp for additional benefit.

Shampoos containing biotin, silica, aloe vera gel, vitamins C and E, and jojoba oil are all very good for the hair. Do not use cheap, grocery store variety shampoos and conditioners. They contain toxic chemicals that not only can damage the hair, but may cause numerous health problems. Look for products without propylene glycol or sodium laurel sulfate.

Crash dieting can ultimately lead to hair loss because of a lack of dietary protein and resulting nutritional deficiencies.

ACTION PLAN FOR HEALTHY HAIR
GENERAL RECOMMENDATIONS

- Use only natural hair products free of harsh chemicals and additives. Brush your hair often with a natural bristle brush, making sure to work the scalp well.

DIETARY TIPS

- Eat foods rich in biotin and inositol, including brewer's yeast, brown rice, green peas, lentils, oats, walnuts, sunflower seeds, and supplements. Follow a whole-food diet. Also include essential fatty acids (EFAs) in the form of wild salmon or nuts and seeds. EFAs are also available in capsule form through healthtreasurechest.com. Go to products and supplements.

BENEFICIAL VITAMINS, MINERALS, AND HERBS

Silica— Is one of the most abundant minerals in the world; it is found in all connective tissues, including hair. It strengthens and prevents hair loss. Food sources are seafood, rice, soybeans, and green vegetables. One of the best dietary sources of silica is whole grain products.

Horsetail— Is an herb that is a rich source of silica. Horsetail can be found in natural food stores and can be found in the form of tea, tinctures, or capsules.

Inositol and **Choline**— Are two of the lesser-known nutrients that can improve hair health. Numerous supplement combinations are available in health food stores that contain these two, plus all the nutrients needed for healthy hair.

GET HEALTHY, AMERICA!

HAIR-BUILDING FRESH JUICE

Healthy Hair Drink
    1 stalk of celery
    1 handful mixed leafy greens
    1 carrot
    ½ lemon, peeled
    1 handful parsley
    ¼ small beet
    ½ apple
    Piece of raw ginger the size of a quarter

*   Push through a juicer and drink immediately.

1 5 The Fingernails

Fingernails can be an indicator of a person's health status. Some researchers feel that what you see on the outside is a reflection of what's going on inside. Fingernail problems may be due to poor nutrition, confirms James Balch, M.D., in his best-selling book, *Prescription for Nutritional Healing*. He describes several clues the fingernails can give:

- A lack of protein, folic acid, and vitamin C causes hangnails. White bands across the nails are also an indication of protein deficiency. Insufficient amounts of complete proteins and/or vitamin A slows down growth.
- A lack of vitamin A and calcium causes dryness and brittleness.
- A lack of the B vitamins causes fragility, with horizontal and vertical ridges.
- Hangnails may result from inadequate vitamin C, B vitamins (especially folic acid), and protein.
- Insufficient intake of vitamin B12 leads to excessive dryness, very rounded and curved nail ends, and darkened nails.
- An iron deficiency may result in "spoon" nails (nails that develop a concave shape) and/or vertical ridges.
- Zinc deficiency may cause the development of white spots on the nails.
- A lack of sufficient "friendly" bacteria (lactobacilli) in the body can result in the growth of fungus under and around the nails.
- A lack of sufficient hydrochloric acid (HCl) contributes to splitting nails.[70]

ACTION PLAN FOR HEALTHY NAILS
GENERAL RECOMMENDATIONS

- Whether you want your nails to show signs of a healthy body or just want them to be strong and pretty, following a whole-food, natural diet is a starting point. Including plenty of raw fruits, vegetables, raw nuts, and seeds is an excellent way to guarantee that you are getting the nutrition you need.

DIETARY TIPS

- Avoid refined foods, as they lack nutrients.

- Make sure you are getting ample protein in the form of lean meats, chicken, fish, or vegetable sources such as nuts and seeds.

- Eat plenty of foods rich in the B vitamin biotin: brewer's yeast, soy, and whole grains.

- Eat foods rich in sulfur and silicon: broccoli, fish, onions, sea vegetables, and drink horsetail tea.

- Include calcium-rich foods daily: sesame seeds, cheese, salmon, blackstrap molasses, almonds, and dark and leafy-green vegetables.

GET HEALTHY, AMERICA!

HEALTHY FINGERNAIL JUICE

Strong-As-Nails Delight
    2 kale leaves
    1 handful spinach
    1 handful leafy greens such as Swiss chard, kale and romaine
    1 small apple

- Push through a juicer and drink immediately.

NUTRITION FOR COMMON AILMENTS

1 6 Acne to Edema

Long before we "moderns" frequented the planet, foods and herbs were regarded as potent medicine. With the onset of the modern pharmaceutical industry and prescription drugs, we lost the knowledge of how to use natural remedies—something our ancestors learned over time through trial and error.

Science is now confirming that many of these folk remedies have distinct pharmacological properties proven to be just as valuable today as they were generations ago. What's more, they are generally inexpensive, harmless, and effective!

When I was a child in the 1950s, there were a few drugs available, albeit not many (and for sure, they had far fewer side effects). Our medicine cabinet always had Vicks Vapor Rub for colds, Absorbine Junior for sore muscles, Noxema for sunburns, zinc oxide ointment for burns, and iodine or mecurachrome for cuts. If we got the flu, my mom would take us to see dear old Dr. Friedland for a shot of penicillin.

However, my grandma Jessie and my aunt Bessie were always ready to fix whatever ailed us with things from the kitchen. If it was a cold, they would reach for the brown jar of rendered goose fat and rub it on our chests. Then they would pin a flannel cloth to the inside of our pajama tops before they bedded us down for the night. The goose fat had been rendered from the Christmas goose, mixed with Minard's linament, and stored in jars. (Minard's linament, a bit of American nostalgia, was a menthol product.) It always seemed to help—and memories of their loving care have stuck with me a lifetime!

The list of conditions below is not inclusive, and there are dozens of other remedies that might be just as effective. Check the book list for additional reading material on natural cures.

The remedies suggested here are strictly informational and never a replacement for qualified medical attention. Always seek a professional opinion for any serious health issue and use only under a doctor's advice if you are pregnant or taking prescription medication.

ACNE

- A diet low in zinc may promote acne. Zinc-rich foods include herring, wheat germ, sesame seeds, blackstrap molasses, sunflower seeds, whole-grains, and raw nuts.

- Acidophilus, used as directed on the label, repopulates the colon with friendly bacteria and keeps the bad bacteria at bay.

- Acne can result from food allergies or sensitivities. Get an examination by a healthcare practitioner or do home testing to determine what foods may be affecting you negatively. Foods high on the allergic list include milk, wheat, eggs, peanuts, sugar, soy, and chocolate. Go to healthtreasurechest.com and the Food Sensitivity Testing tab for information.

- Beneficial cleansing herbs (can be used topically or orally): ginger, aloe, garlic, cascara sagrada, dandelion, and alfalfa.

- Beneficial nutrients include vitamin A, niacin, zinc, and MSM (do not use if sulfur sensitive).

- Drink at least eight glasses of pure water daily. Make sure your water is pure.

- Eat chlorophyll-rich green foods for their detoxifying benefits: all dark leafy-green vegetables and powdered green foods like barley green, algae/seaweed, liquid chlorophyll, or fresh wheatgrass juice.

- Eat more raw foods of dark color like beets, berries, dark and leafy greens, red grapes, and broccoli. Also include raw nuts and seeds.

- Maintain a fiber-rich diet to keep the colon clear. Remove all white-flour products from the diet.

- Remove all sugar and products with sugar from the diet.

- Use only hormone-free meat and dairy products. Find an organic supplier.

- Don't use commercial soaps. Buy and use naturally made varieties that are free of chemicals.

APPENDICITIS

- Eat a high-fiber diet rich in whole-grains, fruits, and vegetables. Fiber helps move food through the intestines and helps avoid a back-up into the appendix. Often a forerunner to colon disease, which may show later in life, appendicitis is usually a result of poor elimination.[71]

ATHLETE'S FOOT

- Colloidal silver applied topically, as directed on label, works as a natural antibiotic, destroying fungi, viruses, and bacteria. Available through *www.gethealthyamerica.biz.*

- Cut sugar out of the diet because it feeds the fungus.

- Dust feet with garlic powder.

- Olive-leaf extract, oregano oil, or tea tree oil rubbed on the area may benefit.

- Probiotics—friendly bacteria like acidopholis—can be taken in oral form to implant the colon with the proper balance of bacteria. Having the correct amount internally will aid in control of external manifestations of fungal overgrowth like athlete's foot.

- Soak feet in two-parts vinegar and one-part warm water several minutes daily until symptoms are relieved. If itching begins again, immediately re-start the vinegar wash. Apply pure olive oil after treatment and wear socks morning and evening.

- Soak feet in hydrogen peroxide (3% strength) or dab it on affected areas with a cotton ball.

BEDWETTING

- Check for food allergies and sensitivities. Go to the Food Sensitivity Testing Tab at healthtreasurechest.com for information.

- My oldest son was a bedwetter, long before I knew anything about nutrition. I purchased a program that used an alarm. It went off the second he started to wet the bed. It worked, and quickly! Check the internet under enuresis.

- The herbs buchu, corn silk, and parsley, taken as tea before dinner so they have time to work and be eliminated before bedtime, have been reported to be beneficial.

BEE STING

- Vitamin C rub: Mix powdered vitamin C with a few drops of water to make a thick paste, remove stinger, and cover the sting area immediately with the rub. The same procedure also applies to non-poisonous spider bites. It may be beneficial to take oral vitamin C, up to 1000 mg. every hour for a few hours.

BLADDER INFECTION

- Bucha herb tea helps relieve the burning sensation on urination.
- Cranberry juice (sugar-free) acidifies the urine and inhibits bacterial growth.
- D-mannose found in natural supplements for the bladder keeps the bacteria down in the bladder. (See kidneys in index.)
- Fresh blueberries have anti-bacterial properties and are cleansing to the bladder.
- Parsley tea keeps urine flowing, to help flush the bladder.
- Vitamin C taken by mouth has antibacterial affects by acidifying the urine.

BRUISING

- Chronic bruising should always be evaluated by a physician.
- Beneficial foods and juices include kale, parsley, broccoli, and green pepper for vitamin C.

- Bioflavonoids work together with vitamin C to strengthen capillaries. Available in supplemental form, it is also in the white lining of oranges and grapefruits.

- Vitamin E applied topically may speed healing. Vitamin E is available in liquid or capsule form. Pop a capsule open and rub the contents on the bruise.

MINOR BURNS

- Aloe Vera rubbed on topically provides relief and speeds healing of minor "household" burns. Keep an aloe plant in your house for various uses.

MY "CURLING IRON STORY"

"I COULD TELL IT WAS GOING TO BE PAINFUL"

"Recently, my curling iron broke. As it did, I ended up with a rather severe burn on the palm of my right hand. I could tell that it was going to be painful, so I went to the organic garden at the Optimum Health Institute (where I was staying for an extended period in 2007) and broke off a piece of an aloe vera plant growing there. I immediately rubbed the burn thoroughly with the sticky liquid inside the plant. It did such an excellent job that I didn't have one bit of pain after that."

CANCER

This topic will require major research on your part. If you are seeking alternative approaches, you will find numerous clinics worldwide that work with natural therapies. The Gerson Institute and the Oasis of Hope are examples. Find out what is available that will enhance any other treatments you are receiving from your doctor. Alternative therapies can include (but are not limited to) wheatgrass juice, large quantities of raw vegetable juices, coffee enemas, an all-raw diet, and much more.

CANKER SORES

- Acidophilus found in yogurt or available in capsules will help balance intestinal flora.

- Nutritional yeast is high in the B vitamins, which help stop canker sores. It is excellent when added to smoothies and is available in natural food stores.

- Canker sores often indicate a vitamin C deficiency; supplementation may be beneficial.

- Herbs: Goldenseal and sage can be taken in teas, tinctures, or dabbed directly on the sore.

- Test for food allergies or sensitivities. Remove any offending foods. I used to keep dehydrated pineapple on hand for snacks. Later, my oldest son, who couldn't stay out of it, determined it gave him canker sores. Tomatoes also caused him a problem.

- Maintain a diet high in fresh fruits and vegetables to keep the body alkaline.

- Rinse your mouth with sodium ascorbate. Dissolve a spoonful in one half cup water and hold in the mouth for a few seconds.

- Rub vitamin E on the sores several times daily.

CROHN'S DISEASE

- Suggested reading: *Breaking the Vicious Cycle* by Elaine Gottschall. This book suggests removing all grains from the diet, particularly grains with gluten (wheat, rye, oat, and barley). *The Maker's Diet* by Dr. Jordan Rubin. Dr. Rubin cured himself of Crohn's disease with raw foods and fermented foods, as well as use of a special probiotic formulation. Check the web for information about these books.

EAR INFECTION OR ACHE

- Buy garlic oil or make your own by heating a few bulbs in olive oil. Cool, then filter the oil and place a drop in the ear.

- Warm three cloves of garlic and mash. Put in a piece of cloth and place over the painful ear.

EDEMA (WATER RETENTION)

- Eat more potassium-rich foods such as garlic, figs, brown rice, apricots, spinach, yams, and bananas.

- Eliminate condiments high in sodium.

- Make a freshly prepared juice from dandelion greens, cucumbers, and celery.

- Parsley tea taken several times a day is a natural diuretic and may be beneficial.

- Drink plenty of water to flush the system of toxins. Divide your body weight in half and take that number in ounces daily.

🅑🅼 Fractures to Nosebleeds

FRACTURES

If you have a removable cast, a comfrey poultice might help. Use dried or fresh comfrey, roots and leaves if possible. Make a poultice from cheesecloth or other material with the comfrey inside (like a giant, medicated bandage). Wet thoroughly with warm water to activate the components of the comfrey. Place the poultice over the injured area several times daily (American Indians called comfrey "knitbone"). This may be used, along with regular medical treatment such as removable casts and ace bandages, as prescribed by your doctor.

ELIZABETH BAKER ON COMFREY AND FRACTURES
"I WAS UP IN THREE WEEKS INSTEAD OF SIX!"

"In 1995, I was teaching a raw-food preparation class for the National Health Federation in L.A. I was on a platform that wasn't flush to the wall, and when I stepped backward, I fell off the platform and broke my back. My doctor told me that I would be in bed for six weeks. I had comfrey in my yard, so I had my helpers make and apply a comfrey poultice to the injured area several times a day. I was up in three weeks rather than six."[72]

GALLSTONES

Dr. Jonathan Wright M.D., writes:
> According to James C. Breneman, M.D., past chairman of the Food Allergy Committee of the American College of Allergists,

gallbladder attacks could be completely avoided by eliminating allergic foods from the diet. He took sixty-nine patients who had gallbladder pain and put them on a diet of foods he felt had minimum allergic potential—beef, rye, rice, and spinach. He reported that, 'All the patients (100%) were relieved of their symptoms at the end of one week's use of the basic elimination diet.' It usually took three to five days for their symptoms to disappear.[73]

- See the section on digestion in this book for gallbladder cleanses. Do any cleanse under the direction of a healthcare practitioner.

- Lecithin, a fat emulsifier, aids digestion of fats and helps prevent the formation of gallstones. A granule form is available in natural food stores and can be added to smoothies.

- The herb alfalfa cleanses the gallbladder and supplies nutrients. Take as a supplement or a tea.

GOUT

- Gout usually occurs in overweight people and in those who indulge in rich foods and alcohol; typically attacks joints in hands and feet, particularly the big toe; deposits of crystallized uric acid cause swelling and severe pain.

- Celery seeds help stimulate the elimination of uric acid. A tea made from two teaspoons celery seed in one cup of water can be used two times a day. Also eat fresh celery.

- Drink water freely—divide your body weight in half and drink that many ounces daily.

- Eat a low-purine diet. High-purine foods should be entirely omitted. Purine-containing foods include beer and other alcoholic beverages, anchovies, sardines, fish roe, herring, yeast, and organ meat (liver, kidneys, sweetbreads, consommé, and gravies).

- Get off all junk food, including refined carbohydrates: candy, cookies, pastas, doughnuts, etc. Focus on a low-fat diet—no fried foods, greasy meals, etc.

- Noni juice, a favorite of the Polynesians, is said to relieve gout. Available in natural food stores.

- Eat cherries or drink cherry juice daily during an attack. Dr. Blau certainly found relief from this tasty fruit:

DR. BLAU'S CHERRY STORY

"EAT CHERRIES EVERY DAY DURING AN ATTACK!"

Ludwig W. Blau, PhD, discovered how cherries could help gout. Crippled and in a wheelchair, he was hungry so wheeled himself to the kitchen. Finding nothing interesting in the cupboards, he opened the refrigerator and saw a bowl of cherries, which he ate. The next morning, the pain and inflammation in his toes had nearly disappeared.

He had remembered his doctor telling him to eat foods low in purines. This included cherries. His doctor also suggested that he avoid foods such as anchovies, bouillon, herring, meat extracts, organ meats, and sardines.

He decided to eat at least six cherries a day and was soon out of his wheelchair. He was so much better, he was able to go back to normal activity levels.

On a business trip a while later, he forgot to bring his cherry supply. Very quickly, this led to his discovery that the pain had returned and his toes once again were throbbing with pain. He resumed eating cherries and, in only a few days, his gout diminished again.

Blau's doctor listened to what Blau had to say and subsequently tried it on twelve of his gout patients. All of those patients improved by eating cherries or drinking cherry juice.

HEADACHE & MIGRAINES

- Chamomile herb tea is helpful in relaxing muscles.

- Eliminate foods containing the amino acid tyramine (bananas, chicken, chocolate, citrus, dairy products, onions, and peanuts). Check the internet for more foods with tyramine.

- Feverfew herb combats inflammation and has been shown to relieve headaches in numerous studies. This herb is available in many natural food stores. Do not use when pregnant.

- Headaches may be an allergic reaction to wheat, MSG, sulfites, sugar, hot dogs, lunch meats, dairy products, nuts, citric acid, cheese, sour cream, yogurt, alcohol, vinegar, or marinated foods. See allergy section for more information on testing for allergies.

- The herb cayenne thins the blood and may reduce pain by keeping the blood flowing smoothly. Various forms of this herb can be found in natural food stores.

- Magnesium supplementation may be beneficial for migraine headaches, as the following two stories show. Magnesium/calcium supplements are available in natural food stores. Jay S. Cohen, M.D., says that,

My own migraines disappeared (except for an occasional painless, visual aura) since I began taking magnesium. It is far safer, cheaper, and often more effective than many expensive, side-effect prone drugs.[74]

ROBIN'S STORY

"I WOULDN'T WISH THOSE MIGRAINES ON MY WORST ENEMY"

Robin is my tax accountant. We were talking one afternoon when I stopped in to pick up my taxes. Knowing that I was writing a book about natural health, she told me that she had suffered beyond belief with migraines for many years. She had a migraine almost every week; each would last for three days.

"When the migraine finally would go away, it would take me the rest of the week to totally recover," she told me. "So I did some deductive reasoning and research. I remembered that when I was pregnant, they gave me magnesium sulfate to slow down my uterine contractions.

Then I read that veins have smooth muscles around them, so I wondered if magnesium might relax the veins in my head when I had a migraine. Better yet, I wondered if it might stop them before they happened. So I bought a calcium/magnesium supplement at the health food store and started taking the recommended amount.

I am here to tell you that my migraines have gone away! Sometimes I get just a twinge of pain during my period, but it never lasts and never develops into a migraine. My doctor later apologized to me and said he simply wasn't taught anything about nutrition in medical school!"

INSOMNIA

- Magnesium and calcium supplementation at bedtime may be beneficial. Supplements are available in natural food stores.

- Shut out all light while sleeping. Sleeping in a dark room aids production of the neurotransmitter *serotonin*, which is crucial in making melatonin, the "sleep" hormone.

- The following herbs may be beneficial taken as a tea prior to bed: peppermint, kava kava, lemon balm, valerian root, catnip, and chamomile.

- Tryptophan-rich foods can make you sleepy if eaten two hours prior to bedtime: turkey, bananas, dates, figs, nut butter, and yogurt.

- Avoid foods that contain the amino acid tyramine, which increases norepinephrine, a brain stimulant: bacon, cheese, chocolate, eggplant, ham, potatoes, sauerkraut, sugar, spinach, tomatoes, and wine.

MULTIPLE SCLEROSIS

- Have testing for allergies and sensitivities to foods and chemicals. Remove allergens from diet and environment.

- Eat a whole food diet with plenty of raw fruits and vegetables.

- Research the topic of mercury toxicity and removal of amalgam fillings.

- The book we referred people to at the Tahoma Clinic was, *The Multiple Sclerosis Diet Book: a Low-Fat Diet for the Treatment of M.S.* by Roy L. Swank. There have been several other good books published since then, available on the internet and in bookstores.

- Use organically grown foods with no chemicals.

NOSEBLEED

Always see a healthcare professional for persistent nosebleeds, as they may indicate a more serious problem.

- Avoid foods high in salicylates (aspirin-like substances) found in apricots, almonds, cherries, currants, plums, mint, oil of wintergreen, and tomatoes.

- Frequent nosebleeds may indicate a vitamin K deficiency. Add vitamin K foods such as alfalfa, kale, and all dark and leafy-green vegetables.

- Frequent nosebleeds may also indicate a vitamin C deficiency. Adding vitamin C with bioflavonoids may promote healing. Foods sources include grapefruits, oranges, and horsetail tea.

- Saturate a piece of cloth in ice water, put above upper teeth against gums or the bridge of the nose, and hold a few moments.

18 Periodontal Disease to Warts

PERIODONTAL DISEASE

- Aloe Vera rubbed on gums or gargled is very healing; keep an aloe vera plant in the bathroom. Aloe is available in natural food stores.

- Vitamin C builds collagen. In one major study, as little as 60 mg a day of vitamin C began to rebuild the gums. First, the subjects were deprived of vitamin C. Later, the subjects took supplements of 60 to 70 mg (the amount in just one orange). The subjects' bleeding gums decreased, white-blood cell formation increased, collagen producing fibroblasts increased, and the gums showed signs of better health. [75]

SHIN SPLINTS

- A poultice (like a giant bandage) made from the herb comfrey applied to the tender area 2–3 times daily for a few minutes may help the inflammation of the legs. See herb section for directions on making a poultice (this worked very well for my youngest son when he ran track in high school).

SINUSITIS

- Gingerroot, crushed and applied as a poultice to the forehead and nose, will stimulate circulation and drainage. Drinking ginger tea can also help clear the sinuses.

- Horseradish, taken as strong as possible (with food or alone), helps open sinuses.

- Food sensitivity testing may be beneficial. Suspect foods include dairy, wheat, eggs, and soy.

- A professor of medicine at UCLA found, by reading early medical literature, that foods used centuries ago to relieve respiratory diseases are quite similar to current day drugs. The common action is to thin out and help move the lung's secretions so they do not clog air passages. Called "mucokinetic" (mucus moving) agents, they help the body to cough up or expel the mucus. They include such food items as the chili pepper and hot, pungent foods. Along this line, Hippocrates prescribed vinegar and pepper to relieve respiratory infections.[76]

SORE THROAT/COUGH

- German doctors commonly recommend a hot-sage gargle for sore throat and tonsillitis. Use one to two teaspoons of fresh (or dried) sage leaves per cup of boiling water. Steep ten minutes. Don't give medicinal doses of sage to children under the age of two.

ALEC'S STORY

"I LOVE YOU DEARLY, BUT THAT NAGGING COUGH IS DRIVING ME CRAZY"

When he was in sixth grade, my youngest son had an irritating cough that held on after a bout of the flu. He was on the mend, but was left with one of those nagging dry throats that caused him to hack about every thirty seconds. It went on for a couple days. It was that kind of cough that drives you around the bend! I knew he couldn't help it, but the hacking was more than any of us could stand.

I found an herbal recipe that I've now used for years. I had all the ingredients in the cupboard, so I made it for him.

I took a cup of the mix and a spoon to the family room where he was and said, "I love you dearly, but that nagging cough is driving me crazy. Take a spoonful of this every fifteen minutes or whenever you feel like coughing."

He did as I said, and like magic, his cough calmed down for the first time in days. After a few minutes, when he felt like coughing again, he would take another spoonful. This little formula worked better than all the cough syrups I'd brought home. Since that experience, I've given my children (even as adults) the simple, safe formula dozens of times and have shared it with anyone interested. Here it is:

The "Can't Stand That Cough" Recipe
¼ teaspoon ginger
¼ teaspoon cayenne
1 tablespoon honey
1 tablespoon vinegar
1 tablespoon hot water to dissolve

- Take a spoonful when coughing occurs and repeat as often as needed.

ULCERS

- Licorice (DGL) in chewable tablets can help protect the digestive tract. DGL licorice has had the glycyrrhizin removed so it can be safely used without worry of elevating the blood pressure or causing water retention. Many studies suggest that DGL may be beneficial in treating peptic ulcers.

- Stop eating foods to which you are allergic (Go to Food Sensitivity Testing at healthtreasurechest.com).

- The herbs slippery elm and marshmallow may be soothing when taken as a supplement.

- Traditionally, raw cabbage juice has been used for stomach ulcers. In the 1950s, Dr. Garnett Cheney of Stanford's School of Medicine, found that raw cabbage juice taken daily was highly beneficial.[77]

VARICOSE VEINS

- A deficiency of vitamin C and bioflavonoids can weaken the collagen structure in the vein walls. Vitamin C and bioflavonoid-rich foods include peppers, buckwheat, currants, grapes, elderberries, hawthorn berry, horsetail, and the white lining of citrus fruits.

- Constipation and downward pressure while evacuating can make varicose veins worse. Ensure that you are getting plenty of dietary fiber to avoid constipation.

- Herbs with known benefits include witch hazel and butcher's broom. Available in several forms in natural food stores.

WARTS

If you've seen a doctor and had warts removed, only to have them grow back, you might try one of these folk remedies. Though these remedies may sound very unscientific and a little like hocus-pocus, I have included them because I've seen most of them work.

- An old Indian method that is said to work well is to pick a dandelion two or three times a day and put the milk from the cut end on the wart. The warts are said to be gone in no time, and they don't grow back as they can after having them burned off.

- Apply castor oil on the wart every day until it's gone. Cover with a bandage.

- Crush a garlic clove, apply directly to the wart, cover with a bandage, and leave on for twenty-four hours. Repeat until wart disappears.

- Mix equal parts lavender, tea-tree oil, and lemon oil. Place a small amount on a bandage and cover the wart. Replace the bandage daily. Continue such treatment until the wart is gone.

- Squeeze the contents of a vitamin E capsule directly on the wart and cover with a bandage—continue for one to three weeks or until the wart is gone (read Rodney's story; see index).

- The milky juice of fresh figs applied directly on warts several times a day for a couple weeks may be effective.

ALLERGIES- EATING OURSELVES SICK!

1 9 Eating Ourselves Sick!

BENJAMIN'S STORY

"AT OUR HOUSE, MILK IS LIKE ARSENIC "

Carol Nelson is afraid of cheese, milk, and anything else that comes from a cow. It is an odd phobia, but Carol has every reason to fear dairy products. Her son Benjamin nearly died from eating a slice of Swiss cheese.

"At our house, milk is like arsenic," she said. "When Benjamin was ten months old, I gave him a piece of Swiss cheese, and he went in to anaphylaxis. He couldn't breathe, and his face swelled. When we got him to the hospital, they told me he had allergies." (Anaphylaxis is a life threatening reaction to a specific substance.) Milk turned out to be just one of several severe allergies Benjamin had. Benjamin is also allergic to eggs and peanuts. He is four now and still not able to eat these foods.

———

While anaphylaxis is rarely seen in a clinical setting (these people usually end up in the emergency room), as the clinical nutritionist at the Tahoma Clinic, I saw my share of less reactive allergies—let's call them sensitivities—to all sorts of foods and environmental toxins. According to the National Institute of Allergy and Infectious Diseases, serious allergies/sensitivities affect more than 50 million Americans.[78]

WHAT IS AN ALLERGY?

Most of us recognize seasonal allergies, but we are less familiar with food allergies. Also called *food intolerances* (or *food sensitivities*), testing for them was a common procedure at the Tahoma Clinic. Numerous patients made their way down the hall to the allergy department, orders in hand, because the doctor suspected foods (or common environmental chemicals) were contributing to their health issues.

When Dr. Wright sent my five-year-old son Jake down that hall in years past, he was pretty sure how the testing would come out.

JAKE'S STORY

"MOM, MY BRAIN SEEMS TO FUNCTION BETTER NOW"

Long before I worked at the Tahoma Clinic with Dr. Wright, I began studying food allergies, and I soon noticed that my five-year-old son had signs and symptoms that closely paralleled what I'd been reading about.

I had read Dr. Wright's column, "Mailbag," in *Prevention* magazine. He wrote one month on food allergies and sensitivities, so I made an appointment for Jake as the clinic was just thirty minutes up the road.

As a child, Jake's cheeks were often ruddy with small bumps and his pupils were frequently dilated. He was an extremely busy child, bordering on what today would be called hyperactivity.

On appointment day with Dr. Wright, we completed the initial check-in procedures with the nurse and were escorted to an examination room. Dr. Wright's nurse reassured me by saying, "Dr. Wright will figure out what's wrong with your son."

Dr. Wright entered the room and began the exam. Almost immediately, stethoscope pressed against Jake's chest, he said, "This child has allergies." He pointed out his allergic shiners (dark circles under the eyes) and Dennie's lines (horizontal creases under the eyes.) So Jake was sent for food allergy testing.

During Jake's testing, each food or chemical suspected of causing the reaction was injected just under the skin and physical reactions were recorded. After about ten minutes, a neutralizing dose was given to stop any symptoms that had been evoked. His treatment included oral neutralizing drops.

Over several weeks of testing, Jake was checked on wheat, eggs, corn, peanuts, chicken, beef, and numerous household chemicals. He didn't react in an unusual way. Soy would be a different story!

As a child, Jake was allergic to cow's milk, so I substituted soy milk. On soy day, the nurse gave him the injection and he returned to his seat next to me. Almost instantly, he began to rock, almost as though he was on a rocking horse—back and forth, back and forth! I watched in disbelief.

Soy was the only food to which he visibly reacted—the very food that was a diet basic for him. When the neutralizing dose was given, he returned to his normal self.

One day, when Jake and I were at the clinic, a woman named Linda was in to be tested on numerous chemicals she was exposed to at work. After her injection, she returned to her chair, face cupped in hands. Soon, she began sobbing—uncontrollably! Because of her behavior, I first thought that someone had said something unkind to her.

A few minutes later, she took the neutralizing dose and quickly returned to her normal self. Unexplained crying was the reason she came to the Tahoma Clinic.

This was my first experience with food and chemical sensitivities. In later years, as the clinical nutritionist at the Tahoma Clinic, I found that these reactions were not unusual at all! All too frequently, symptoms like her crying or Jake's rocking were blamed on things like being neurotic, having ADHD, or having no discipline at home.

My son Jake got better when we eliminated the soy (wheat and milk also) from his diet. A few months later, he said, "Mom, my brain seems to function better now."

FOOD SENSITIVITY & INTOLERANCE

An allergic response (allergy) or food sensitivity is an inappropriate reaction by the body's immune system to a food or substance that is not normally considered harmful. The immune system tries to fight off the substance with responses like nasal congestion, coughing, wheezing, shortness of breath, indigestion, headache, fatigue, hives, skin rashes, and more.

A reaction may begin as soon as a person starts chewing food (I've even seen people who begin to sneeze when they just peel potatoes, onions, or other foods). Or symptoms can manifest within two to forty-five minutes or longer. Each person is individual. Reactions are also known to occur as far out as three or four days. These delayed reactions are more difficult to identify since most of us don't remember what we ate three days ago. Arthritic aches and pains, or constipation and diarrhea, can be delayed reactions. Symptoms caused from sensitivities are not usually life threatening.

WHAT ARE SOME SYMPTOMS AND THEIR CAUSES?

As the clinical nutritionist at the Tahoma Clinic a decade, I saw my share of patients with food and environmental allergies. The symptoms were diverse and many, including:

Abnormal body order

Acne

Arthritis

Asthma

Bedwetting

Bulimia

Colitis

Conjunctivitis

Depression

Ear infections

Eczema

Excessive perspiration

Eye pain

Fatigue

Headaches

Hives

Hyperactivity

Learning disorders

Migraines

Obesity

Respiratory infections

Restless legs

Skin rashes

POSSIBLE FOODS AND CHEMICALS THAT CAN CAUSE REACTIONS INCLUDE:

Beef

Certain metals

Chicken

Cleaning supplies

Corn
Cosmetics
Dairy
Dust
Dust mites
Eggs
Insect venoms
Lanolin
Laundry softener
Mold
Oranges
Peanuts
Pollen
Soap
Soy
Wheat

Keep in mind these are just examples. Any food or chemical can cause a reaction in susceptible people. In years past, my husband developed an itch that almost drove him crazy, and he tried to continue working with that terrible itch. We finally pinpointed the culprit to be a laundry softener I had been using. The itching stopped when I discontinued using it.

Clearly, not all problems can be blamed on allergies or sensitivities. But it is a good idea to consider them as a piece of the puzzle if you are trying to solve a riddle of unexplained illness.

HOW TO TEST FOR ALLERGIES OR SENSITIVITIES

Testing in a Clinical Setting: Several methods are used in medical clinics to test for allergies or sensitivities. According to the American Academy of Family Physicians:

> There are three main kinds of skin tests. The first kind is called a "scratch" or a "prick" test. A tiny drop of testing fluid is placed on the skin. Then, the skin is pricked through the drop. After 15 minutes, the test site is checked for redness and swelling. There's a "prick" sensation when the testing is applied, but it doesn't hurt a lot. Usually, about 40 prick tests are needed for a full exam.
>
> In the second kind of skin test, the testing fluid is injected into the skin (like a shot). This test is used to check for allergy to medicines (most often penicillin) and bee-sting allergy.
>
> The third kind of skin test is called a patch test. A small patch of material, soaked in testing fluid, is taped on your skin. After two or three days, your doctor will take off the patch and look for redness and swelling on your skin. Patch tests are used to evaluate rashes caused by allergy to things that might rub against your skin.[79]

Pulse Testing: This testing is done at home. Dr. Arthur Coca discovered that a person's pulse will rise after exposure to an allergenic substance. He published a layman's version of his concepts in *The Pulse Test.* If you suspect you are reacting to a certain food or chemical that you use frequently, a simple pulse test can help you solve the mystery.

The pulse testing involves taking a resting pulse, eating a certain food, or being exposed to a particular substance, and then taking the pulse again after thirty minutes. A decrease or increase in pulse rate indicates a sensitivity to the substance being tested. You will want to take a resting pulse before you begin the test.

Sit quietly for ten minutes, then take your pulse. When testing foods, eat only one food at a time. Allow one hour before testing the next food or substance. Once you have identified a food or chemical sensitivity, you will want to avoid that item.

Fasting, Followed by Deliberate Food Testing: With this type of testing, three to four days of fasting are undertaken. Then, foods are reintroduced one at a time. During reintroduction, you will note any adverse symptoms. Extended fasting should only be done under the supervision of a qualified healthcare practitioner. See Elizabeth Baker's story of fasting and deliberate food testing found later in this section for a good idea of how this works.

Muscle Testing: Kinesiology means the science of movement. *Applied Kinesiology* was the name given to muscle isolation techniques developed by U.S. chiropractor Dr. George Goodhart.[80] This technique is now used by many alternative chiropractors, osteopaths, medical doctors, dentists, and others with a license to diagnose. Applied Kinesiology is a way to evaluate normal and abnormal body functions by simple muscle testing.

ELIZABETH BAKER WRITES ABOUT MUSCLE TESTING
"HIS ENVIRONMENTAL BIO-WARNING SYSTEM TELLS HIM TO LEAVE IT ALONE"

The sign at the nursery read: Don't compost your potting soil in a plastic container. Smaller print explained the mystery; earthworms can't live in plastic, no matter how well ventilated it is. If they can't escape, they die. By contrast, soil composted in ventilated metal cans offers no problem.

What tells the worm that plastic is poisonous to him? It is the cells of his body. They cannot perform normally because of constant off-gassing of the toxic plastic. His environmental bio-warning system tells him to leave the plastic at once.

In humans this bio-warning mechanism or system is called body language. The body tells what is good or bad for it, not the mind.

The mind is too conditioned—by conscious learning and education, by social and environmental conditioning, by ecological altering of sensory perceptions, by pollution, and by sensitivities both external and ingested—to discern what contact harms or helps.

By a very simple test, the body, without conscious effort of the mind, can indicate what is good and what is bad for it for optimal functioning. To do the test, the person to be tested (the testee) stands and extends the right arm straight out, fist tightly clenched. Test whichever arm is normally used ...if left handed, test left arm; if right handed, test right arm.

The person who does the testing (the tester), with one hand on the testee's wrist, presses down on the extended arm while the testee resists as much as possible. The tester then puts the suspected allergen such as peanut butter, sugar, or chemical substance in the testee's left hand.

Again the testee extends the right arm, makes it rigid, and clenches the fist. The tester presses down on the testee's arm. If the testee's arm is easily forced down despite all efforts to offer as much resistance as in the trial test of strength, the testee is allergic to the item being tested. His body is weakened by contact with the substance. For maximum strength and freedom from the fatigue factor, he should stay away from these items.[81]

ONCE YOU'VE IDENTIFIED OFFENDING ITEMS, TRY A ROTATION DIET

Once you have identified food sensitivities, a rotary-diversified diet referred to here as a rotation diet can be used. Developed by Herbert Rinkel, M.D., it is based on the idea that it takes a food about four days to clear from our systems once we have eaten it. While four days is a standard time, in some people it takes up to ten days until the food components have totally cleared the body.

This is a classic recovery plan, and numerous how-to books have been written on the subject. Some people do well by eliminating any reactive food completely from the diet for a period of ninety days. Others find that they can eat reactive foods only once every four days and do just fine.

As a general rule of thumb, you will eat only specific foods (or foods from specific food families) one day in every four days. For example, it may be beef, rye, and green beans on Monday; chicken, rice, and asparagus on Tuesday; fish, barley, and broccoli on Wednesday; and lamb, oats, and spinach on Thursday. On Friday, you can begin the rotation again. Go to healthtreasurechest.com and the Food Sensitivity Testing tab for information.

Once offending foods are identified then removed, they can usually be added back in time, even tolerated if not eaten too frequently. Elizabeth Baker's road to recovery began with fasting, testing, and a rotation diet plan.

ELIZABETH BAKER BEGINS HER RECOVERY WITH A FOOD-ELIMINATION DIET

"I WAS SO ALLERGIC I SHOULD HAVE BEEN A BUBBLE LADY"

As told by Elizabeth on 10–20–03:
"In 1971, I was so allergic I should have been a bubble lady. Perfume, gas fumes, most foods, and soaps in stores bothered me. I had to stay out of places where these were found. My husband, Elton, would let me out of the car one block before he went into the filling station because of the toxic odor of gasoline.

I was allergic to many foods, but I didn't know it at the time. I could barely function physically—no energy, frequent indigestion, headaches, tremors, shortness of breath, constipation, and dozens of other symptoms. I had been hospitalized and given no hope for my life. Doctors told Elton to check out the mortuary because I would be dead by morning. However, by the grace of God, I was not. I was released to return home, and I decided to call an alternative-therapy physician I had been told about.

The alternate-therapy doctor that I found, dear old Dr. Silver, insisted that I go into a fasting clinic. He and his wife had gone through the clinic before me, and they found out all their allergies through fasting and got over them. I told Dr. Silver that he would have to convince me. Then he'd need to convince my physicist/chemist husband.

The fasting clinic was located in a hospital wing in Coos Bay, Oregon. Elton made me comfortable in the back seat of the car and away we went. I was assigned to a young doctor, Joseph Morgan, M.D. He had studied with the eminent Thereon Randolph, M.D., from Zion International Hospital in Chicago (Dr. Randolph was a pioneering researcher in the area of fasting/testing and food elimination diets to discover allergies). Even though I thought Dr. Silver had lost his marbles to send me off to try fasting, I reasoned that if I was going to die, I might as well die trying.

I was placed on a total fast of water and a bit of salt to keep from dehydrating for eight miserable, miserable days and nights. I had a repeat of every pain, illness, and sickness that I had ever suffered in my life. I had terrible restless legs from my hypoglycemia. Severe agony didn't allow me to sleep but two or three hours a night.

On the eighth day, I woke up feeling great! I could clearly see all the signs across the street. In the woods next door, I could make out the sounds of birds, cracking branches, and animals moving. I made out distinct, separate "woods" sounds. I could touch any fabric or surface and tell what it was—silk, polyester, cotton, linen, nylon, wool, paper, or newsprint. Before, everything felt the same, and I couldn't identify them. I could smell like a bloodhound.

At 10 a.m. on the morning of the eighth day, I was allowed to break the fast (I had asked Dr. Morgan on day five if I could please eat. He said, "Not yet"). I ate an organic banana. No problem. The next morning I had cereal of organic whole wheat cooked only with salt. Feeling good, I took a walk down the hall, then turned around, and headed back toward my room.

There was no one at the nurse's station since it was morning break. Before I could reach my door, I collapsed on the floor. My energy had left as though someone had struck me across the back of the legs. I remember it being the strangest feeling! I just went weak! I crawled to my bed as best I could, but I couldn't get up. A nurse found me lying on the floor soon after and commanded, "Don't move. I am calling the blood man."

The blood man came immediately and drew a sample. Soon he was back with the results. My blood sugar had plunged to an astounding and dangerously low 38! The problem had been the wheat cereal. I was terribly allergic. Wheat also turned out to be the greatest single cause of my aching, fatigue, and low energy.

I stayed in the hospital for two weeks and was tested on thirty-six foods, one at a time and four hours apart. I was allergic to twenty-five out of the thirty-six foods tested and could eat only eleven. I went home with a diet consisting of twelve foods (Dr. Morgan added blueberries, which were not tested but are rarely a problem).

My diet schedule was a single different food for each meal for three meals a day for four days. That gave me all twelve foods. Then, I began the cycle over again. One of the twelve foods was moose meat. My dear husband, Elton, engaged my nephew to go to Canada on an extra hunting trip. He brought me home a moose! The meat was delicious.

Here was my meal plan. On day one, I had three different foods: one for breakfast, one for lunch, and one for dinner. On day two, I had three more foods, following the same pattern as day one. On days three and four, I repeated the pattern, so that by the end of the four days, I had eaten twelve meals, each meal consisting of only one food, and no food was repeated more than once. The foods I could eat were cantaloupe, Brazil nuts, amaranth grain, blueberries, cabbage, raw milk, corn, moose meat, pineapple, apples, bananas, and carrots.

I continued on this rotated diet for a few months, and then slowly began to add other foods. I was feeling great and thought I was essentially well. This is where my personal journey for a disease-free body really began and my calling came from God to tell others about the importance of diet and health. During more than three decades of my journey I have been blessed to recover from three terminal illnesses using natural means and only a small amount of medical intervention."

ALLERGIST DORIS RAPP, M.D., ON ALLERGIES

Doris Rapp, M.D., honored the Get Healthy, America! staff by speaking at one of our seminars in Phoenix in 2003. She is a powerful speaker with an even more powerful message.

As a pediatric allergist, Dr. Rapp specializes in increasing awareness about the potentially tragic, harmful effects of numerous chemicals that we are exposed to on a daily basis. Also working with food allergies as they affect children, she has made videotapes showing their remarkable reactions to certain food.

As the result of her work, she was called late one Tuesday afternoon in 1988 and asked to be a guest on the Phil Donahue Show. She was to bring several mothers and their children, all of whom had been treated at her clinic for food and chemical sensitivities. Five mothers agreed to appear and let their children's videos be shown on national TV.

On the show, a video was shown of a boy who became extremely hyperactive after eating a food to which he was sensitive. As Dr. Rapp wrote in *Is This Your Child?*, "phones rang throughout the country and that show generated over 140,000 letters. Our staff cried on more than one occasion as we read the letters. Many mothers wrote us that tears of joy and relief streamed down their cheeks as they listened to Phil Donahue talk about the unusual types of allergies that could affect some youngsters. They recognized their child."

———

Working for many years at the Tahoma Clinic with Dr. Jonathan Wright, I can confirm, over and over again, that reactions to foods and chemicals can be severe. It was always rewarding to see these children get better by following the plans set out for them by the doctors.

For more information on Food Sensitivity Testing, go to health-treasurechest.com.

HYPOGLYCEMIA AND DIABETES

2 0 Problems of Blood Sugar

The toast pops up, and it sounds like a shotgun firing. She spends two minutes deciding whether to use butter or jam. And when she's finished eating, the dirty plates make her cry. Neurotic? Her husband and doctor think so. But what if they are both wrong?

Her symptoms—sensitivity to slight noise, inability to make decisions, unjustified weeping—are only a few of numerous symptoms that can result from erratic blood sugar. Take Phillip. He would know! His symptoms went far beyond what is considered normal, and an incorrect diagnosis almost cost him his livelihood.

Of the hundreds of clients I worked with at the Tahoma Clinic, Phillip's story would have to be one of the top ten most memorable. Traditional medicine missed the mark by never, ever, asking him about his diet—and a poor diet turned out to be the crux of his problem.

PHILLIP'S STORY
"ALL THEY DID WAS PUT ME ON LIFELONG DISABILITY"

Phillip was a large man, standing over six feet tall and weighing in at 298 pounds. The father of five teenagers, he made his living driving a postal van. In the spring of 1996, he had a sudden onset of seizures, which were accompanied by extreme confusion, shortness of breath, and dizziness. His head would fall backward, and he couldn't speak. When this happened, he said he felt as though he was "going to pass out."

A retired military man, he decided to go for a checkup at the veteran's hospital. After lengthy and intensive examinations with five different specialists, it was decided that Phillip was suffering from what were called *pseudo seizures*—defined as psychogenic nonepileptic seizures—paroxysmal episodes that resemble epileptic seizures; however, they are psychological in origin.[82]

He was placed on lifetime disability and told he should never return to the postal service—that it was dangerous for him to drive. Feeling there was more to his health problems, he decided to visit another local physician. More testing and consultations resulted in the same diagnosis—pseudo seizures.

As a last resort, he called the Tahoma Clinic. It was a miracle that he got a just-cancelled appointment with Dr. Wright, whose schedule was closed. On the day of his appointment, one of the nurses saw him staggering and walking in circles on the sidewalk in front of the clinic. At first, she avoided him thinking he was a drunk, but she ultimately helped him get into the clinic.

After his complete history and physical with the doctor, he saw me. I'll never forget this one—Dr. Wright thought he had Phillip's problem figured out after just talking with him for a few moments. He was right!

"I am retired military—Army—so I went for a checkup since I have the free medical. I had so many tests. They actually sent me to five different specialists."

I asked him about the diagnosis of pseudo-seizures recorded in his chart notes.

"Can you believe it? Pseudo seizures. Like I was making them up!"

Continuing the conversation, I asked, "What were you told to do?"

"They told me I would have to go on lifetime disability, that I could never work again, at least in any job that required driving. Too dangerous! But I have a family to support and almost twenty years in my job. I can't just throw it away! So I made an appointment with this fancy clinic downtown."

"And what did they say?"

"Same story, just several different doctors. They also said I had pseudo seizures."

"Well, it looks like Dr. Wright wants you to have a *six hour glucose tolerance test (GTT).*"

A glucose tolerance test requires that the patient fast overnight, then consume 100-grams of glucose in water. Then blood sugar measurements are taken. Insulin levels may also be measured.

Phillip's chart notes stipulated that the nursing staff was to monitor him closely and stop the test should his symptoms become too severe.

"Let's talk this afternoon, Phillip, after we have the results. And after you've had some lunch."

Several hours later, Phillip was back in my office for a nutritional program. His test was stopped after three hours because he began having the severe reaction Dr. Wright had insisted that the nurses watch for. The results showed that he had extremely erratic blood sugar patterns. I asked him if he knew anything about hypoglycemia, diabetes, or blood sugar.

"Not really. No one ever asked me about that before."

How he could have been seen by that many doctors without any of them questioning him about his diet was beyond me. He'd had a standard blood draw, but there were no red flags. Before we even got into a diet analysis, he said, "I need to tell you that I love sugar! Love it! It is not at all unusual for me to eat a quart of ice cream and four doughnuts for a meal."

Phillip was a very gentle man. He was also honest, sincere, and desperate. We finished his diet history and talked at length about problems of blood sugar. We planned a moderately high-protein, sugar-free, low-carbohydrate meal plan. He would be eating three meals daily with two snacks.

Breakfast included some form of protein like eggs, or cheese; lunch and dinner also had moderate amounts of protein, lots of vegetables, and a small portion of brown rice or potato with skin (to slow down digestion).

Snacks were sugar-free. No more doughnuts and soft drinks, ever! He could eat raw nuts or seeds, low-sugar fruits and nut butter, or cheese and whole-grain crackers.

It is always rewarding to see dramatic results in the healthcare field, but in most cases, health conditions take some time to correct. Phillip was one of those clients who made the job rewarding. Within three days he was a changed man; he returned to work within two weeks.

"I feel wonderful! Look at me! I've done everything you and Dr. Wright asked. No refined sugar at all. And I've eaten consistent meals as you requested. I was able to go back to work in a couple of weeks with no problems!"

Phillip continued with the program that Dr. Wright had ordered, which included nutritional IV therapy, allergy testing, and numerous laboratory tests. And he stayed with his diet plan. About three months later, he was in with his wife. He had lost over fifty pounds! As he sat down in the chair to receive his nutritional IV, his wife looked at me with tears in her eyes.

"I've got my husband back. Thank you all for following your convictions about diet, nutrition, and health. Thank you!"

HYPOGLYCEMIA—UNDER-SWEET BLOOD

Phillip's condition was diagnosed as *hypoglycemia*—an abnormally low level of glucose (sugar) in the blood. Hypoglycemia literally means "under-sweet blood."[83] When Phillip ate too much sugar, the body's response was to trigger the pancreas to pump out insulin; lots of it. This high-octane shot of insulin began to efficiently clear the blood of all that excessive sugar (glucose) from the refined carbohydrates he'd eaten, pushing and storing it in the liver, muscles, and fat cells (Did you hear that? Fat cells).

Phillip's condition, also called *reactive hypoglycemia*, is a medical term defined as occurring two to four hours after a high carbohydrate meal (or oral glucose load). Symptoms include sweating, tremors, rapid heart beat, anxiety and hunger. [84]

What he needed to do was control the amount of glucose (blood sugar) entering his blood by controlling the amount of sugar-laden junk foods that went into his mouth. By stopping all the sugary, highly refined foods and starting on low-sugar foods and unrefined carbohydrates (like beans, whole-grains, and brown rice), he could begin to get control of his blood sugar. This would take the stress off his pancreas by slowing down insulin requirements. In time, over-stimulation of the pancreas can lead to adult onset diabetes as this organ loses its ability to produce the right amounts of insulin.

THE STANDARD AMERICAN DIET & BLOOD SUGAR PROBLEMS

Hypoglycemia is becoming more and more of a problem because of American's poor dietary habits resulting from the Standard American Diet (S.A.D. = sad)—large quantities of simple carbohydrates: candy, soft drinks, all sweets, white-flour pastas, alcohol, pastries, and a huge assortment of processed junk foods.

As early as 1942, the American Medical Association's (AMA) Council on Food and Nutrition made this statement:

> From the health point of view, it is desirable especially to have restriction of such use of sugar as is represented by consumption of sweetened carbonated beverages and forms of candy which are of low nutritional value. The Council believes it would be in the interest of the public health for all practical means to be taken to limit consumption of sugar in any form in which it fails to be combined with significant proportions of other foods of high nutritive quality.[85]

These days, we don't hear much from the AMA of this subject. What started as ten pounds a year per person of sugar in the 1800s has soared to as much as 150 pounds per person today.

And yet, many common conditions result from hypoglycemia: sweating, tremors, anxiety, rapid heartbeat, blurred vision, inability to think/concentrate, light-headedness, fainting spells, craving for sweets, confusion, insomnia, mental disturbances, aggressive behavior, and temper-tantrums.

While the onset of these symptoms may be related to the quality of the meal and/or length of time since the meal, some people don't make that association. Instead, they may grab an aspirin, doughnut, or another cup of coffee—covering up the problem but certainly not correcting it!

DIABETES–A COMMON BLOOD SUGAR PROBLEM

Like hypoglycemia, diabetes is a problem of the pancreas and insulin. *Insulin,* which comes from the pancreas, controls the amount of glucose (sugar) in the blood and the rate at which glucose is absorbed into the cells. In diabetics, glucose builds up in the bloodstream instead of being taken into and used by the cells, leading to abnormally high levels of glucose in the blood. Eventually, this can lead to damaged blood vessels.

There are 20.8 million children and adults in the United States, or 7% of the population, who have diabetes. While an estimated 14.6 million have been diagnosed with diabetes, unfortunately, 6.2 million people (or nearly one-third) are unaware that they have the disease.[86]

There are two major types of diabetes: Type 1 and Type 2. Type 1 usually starts at an early age; the body's immune system attacks and destroys the insulin-producing cells in the pancreas.

Type 2 diabetes is by far the most common form. In Type 2 diabetes, the pancreas does produce insulin in small quantities, but not enough to fuel the cells. The cells may become resistant to the insulin produced, thus resulting in sugar in the blood. Some research has shown that many Type 2 diabetics are actually producing sufficient insulin; however, the cells aren't accepting it.

Type 2 diabetes can be controlled through dietary restrictions. Exercise is also important to keep the blood sugar in control. Combining diet restrictions with a good exercise program can sometimes, eliminate the need for diabetic pills. People who know they have Type 2 diabetes should be under a doctor's care.

Diabetes is out of control in America. Teenagers, and even younger children, are now showing up with Type 2 diabetes. I am amazed at how complacent people have become about having diabetes. It is a serious problem. If you have the diagnosis, you need to take responsibility and make the necessary lifestyle changes to ensure your health.

NEVIN'S STORY, AS TOLD BY RON LOWRIE

"I OFTEN EAT TWO OR THREE BANANAS A DAY"

"Being in pastoral work for over thirty years, it is not unusual to receive phone calls requesting prayer. One came a few years back from a friend named Nevin who had been hospitalized with heart palpitations and intermittent physical weakness. His episodes were coming more and more frequently, yet his physician could find nothing wrong. Because the frequency of the episodes were sporadic, no pattern of occurrence was identified.

I discussed the problem with Nevin, and we prayed. After we hung up, I began thinking about the times we had traveled the freeways together in ministry work decades prior. It was not uncommon for him to eat two to three bananas a day. Raised in the South Pacific, he was accustomed to eating plenty of fruit.

So I called him back and asked him if he was still eating all those bananas. He said yes. I explained the effect of too much sugar (even in fruit) on blood sugar levels, then gave him a glycemic chart that lists the sugar content of various foods. He took it to his doctor who, amazingly, said he'd never seen such a chart.

Nevin stopped eating all the bananas and other sugary food after a little reading on his part, and he had no further bouts with the medically undiagnosed problem."

———

Nevin was getting too much sugar from the bananas and other foods in his diet. Bananas, while a healthy food, are moderately high on the *Glycemic Index*—a scale that ranks carbohydrate-rich foods by how much they raise blood-glucose levels. You will find the Glycemic Index in nutrition books and on the internet.

ACTION PLAN FOR BLOOD SUGAR CONTROL
GENERAL RECOMMENDATIONS

- If you are diabetic and under a doctor's care, be sure to follow the diet instructions given. The following tips may be incorporated when applicable. Dietary alteration is the best way to control any blood sugar problem. Remove all refined sugar from the diet: soft drinks, candy, cookies, pies, cakes, sugary drinks, etc. Stop eating refined, white flour—bread, rolls, pastas, crackers, etc. Find your local health food store and get familiar with all these products made with whole-grains. Also, begin your 10,000-step program and keep at it (see index).

DIETARY TIPS

- Avoid sweet fruit drinks, even 100% pure juice, because of the sugar concentration. Absolutely no soft drinks.

- Don't skip meals; five small meals a day may be helpful in keeping your blood sugar in control (three meals, two snacks).

- Eat ample dietary protein (meat, cheese, eggs, fish, seeds, nuts, tofu, and nut spreads) every day because it digests slowly and stabilizes blood sugar.

- Eat vegetables with skins when possible. The extra fiber will slow down digestion, helping to control blood sugar levels.

- Substitute whole-grain products (including breads, crackers, pastas, muffins, and rolls) for refined grain products.

- Use alcoholic beverages very sparingly if at all.

- Use all fruits in moderation—one to two servings daily. Choose a whole fruit over its juice because the fiber will slow down digestion and slow sugar absorption.

- Use dried fruits, such as raisins and dates, minimally because of the concentrated sugars they contain.

BENEFICIAL VITAMINS, MINERALS, AND HERBS

Chromium Picolinate: A mineral that assists the cells to take in glucose. When chromium is lacking, the effectiveness of insulin is lessened. Chromium should be included in any blood sugar regulation supplement you purchase. Food sources include brewer's yeast, brown rice, cheese, whole-grains, corn, romaine lettuce, onions, and tomatoes.

Cinnamon: Useful for diabetes and blood sugar control. Numerous current studies demonstrate cinnamon's ability to help regulate blood sugar levels. It is now available in capsule form and in combination "blood sugar control" formulations. Sprinkle cinnamon on cereal or bread, stir it into tea, or use as otherwise desired.

Gymnema Sylvestre Leaf (literally means sugar destroyer): Used in the Middle-East for several centuries to regulate sugar. Research has shown that it delays glucose absorption in the intestine. This activity helps prevent the pancreas from releasing too much insulin. The ingredient thought responsible is *gymnemagenin*. The herb is available in capsules.

NATURE'S MOST POWERFUL FOODS

②① Good Fats vs. Bad Fats

In the 1940s and early 1950s, the understanding of scientists was that consuming lots of saturated fats caused atherosclerosis, based on the fact that large amounts of cholesterol were found in atherosclerotic plaques of autopsied persons. From these early observations, scientists created the cholesterol theory. This theory has so inundated the medical community that it's hard to undo that thinking, although "even in the earliest years of research, leading cardiologists strongly resisted the idea that cholesterol was solely responsible for atherosclerosis." [87]

Current studies show that while fats do play a role in the disease, they do not act alone, but rather in concert with other factors, such as a lack of foods high in plant phytochemicals, antioxidants, minerals, and fiber. The pharmaceutical companies tend to ignore this information because it doesn't fit well into "fifteen-second sound bytes on the evening news, or multi-million dollar ad campaigns.[88]

"Unfortunately, modern science, when faced with a paradigm that may endanger funding considerations, tends to ignore such anomalies...."[89]

Despite the ensuing clamor for cholesterol-lowering drugs, studies did not support the theory. In fact, "studies on cholesterol-lowering drugs found no statistical evidence linking reduced cholesterol levels to fewer heart-attack deaths."[90]

STAY AWAY FROM HYDROGENATION & TRANS FATS

Man-made hydrogenated or trans fats are major players on the bad fats team. Hydrogenation is a chemical process that attaches hydrogen to liquid vegetable oil. This action causes the oil to harden, much like lard. Add a little yellow color and butter flavor (after bleaching the mass to hide the horrible smell), and you end up with margarine. I have an old book called *Margarine—the Plastic Fat and Your Heart Attack* by John H. Tobe (1962). He describes how this whole process of hydrogenation damages your arteries and heart. It is out-of-print, but worth a read if you can find it on the internet.[91]

It is now known that hydrogenated or trans fats react negatively in the body and cause cell damage. These damaged cells become sitting ducks; your immune system may then attack them, thinking they are foreign invaders. Many diseases, including cancer and heart disease, have been linked to these artificial fats.

Really, the best way to avoid deadly fats of all types—including those described above—is to stay clear of processed foods. Choose instead whole foods, organic when possible, and the unrefined oils found in health food stores and in the natural food section of your grocery store. These will be labeled as unrefined or will use the terms expeller-pressed, cold-pressed, expeller-processed, or cold-processed.

ESSENTIAL FATTY ACIDS

When you hear "eat good fats," what it usually means is to eat *essential fatty acids* (EFAs)—fat that can't be made by the body. You must eat them in your diet. Eating them is important for healthy hair and skin, to regulate blood pressure and cholesterol, for the production of prostaglandins (important hormone-like messengers), and to help reduce internal inflammation.

EFAs are very important for normal development and function of your brain. Not getting enough can lead to reduced learning ability, depression, and poor recall. There are two important EFAs:

OMEGA-6—LINOLEIC ACID

To get these fats, you will need to eat raw nuts, seeds, legumes, borage oil, grape seed oil, sesame oil and soybean oil. *Omega-6s* are needed for the brain; studies have linked a dietary lack to the development of learning disorders, bipolar disorder disease, Parkinson's disease, and ADD/ADHD, to name a few.

Specifically, cold-water fish has been linked to health for joints, tissues, eyes, hormones, heart, brain, diabetes, cancer, inflammatory bowel disease, and Alzheimer's disease. Because of its powerful anti-inflammatory action, omega-6 can potentially help people suffering from these and other disorders where inflammation plays a role.

OMEGA-3—ALPHA LINOLENIC ACID

Omega-3 fats have been linked to improvement in ADD/ADHD, hyperactivity, aggression, and impulsiveness. They are important for an infant's brain, eye development, and learning ability. To get omega-3, you'll need to eat walnuts, krill oil, cod liver oil, free range eggs, flaxseed oil and cold water fish.

MORE UNHEALTHY FAT

Another issue is one of *interesterified fats*. These fats are fast becoming the method of choice for food manufacturers to replace trans fats because they allow for longer shelf life.

Interesterified fats are oils that have been chemically modified (e.g., turning soybean oil into interesterified soybean oil). This is done in order to make them more solid, less liable to go rancid and more stable for applications such as deep-frying. The interesterification process is used as an alternative to partial hydrogenation, which results in trans fats.[92]

Since we probably won't change or eliminate the fast-food industry—which uses fats to cook the French fries, etc.—it really becomes a personal responsibility to stop eating and feeding deep-fried food to ourselves and those we love.

ACTION PLAN FOR FATS
GENERAL RECOMMENDATIONS

- Eat as much fresh, raw fruits and vegetables as possible. The antioxidants in fruits and vegetables are a major health plus for avoiding artherosclerosis.

- Avoid all types of margarine, shortening, clear liquid (refined oils), lard, and butter substitutes.

- Buy oil in small bottles and refrigerate. Olive oil is the exception and does not need to be refrigerated.

- Don't eat French fries, fried meats, donuts, and other fried foods. Eat only unheated, natural forms of dietary fat like butter, cold-pressed oils, olive oil, nuts, and seeds.

- Eat all fats—even the healthy ones—in moderation (20% to 30% of the diet).

- Eat fast food very, very sparingly, if at all. The huge vats of oil that are used to fry your food are loaded with unhealthy, "oxidized" fats.

- If you are eating fast food, choose from the "healthy" menus that most restaurants now have.

- Eat moderate amounts of raw nuts (not canned, oiled, or salted) for their healthy oil. Always freeze or refrigerate uneaten nuts to preserve health giving properties and stave off rancidity.

- Train your nose to detect rancidity, which is the smell of oil paint (oxidized linseed [flax] oil). Throw out any oils that smell rancid.

- Use coconut oil for high-temperature cooking or red palm oil. Olive oil is a good choice for stir-frying but primarily should be used as a salad dressing or condiment enhancer. Preserving the delicate molecules of olive oil by not using it for high heat cooking is a fundamental health tip for this food spoken of in the Bible.

For important information on fats regarding teens, pregnant women, and children, see the article "Feeding the Next Generation" by Dr. Ellouise Carroll listed later in this book.

22 Fermented Foods— Secret of the Ancients

Fermented foods have been around for centuries and are eaten in Korea (*Kim Chee*), China (*sufu*), Japan (*natto, Miso*), Western cultures (yogurt, *kefir*), Russia (*Kombucha*), and North and Central Europe (*sauerkraut*). Fermentation has been used to enhance the flavor of food and extend shelf life. These cultured foods have always been touted for their health benefits.

THE BENEFITS OF FERMENTED FOODS

During the process of fermentation, microbes break down complex carbohydrates and proteins into more easily digestible elements. There is also an increase of enzymes, which aid digestion and make foods easier to assimilate. Fermented foods colonize the intestinal tract with friendly flora, which help control putrefactive bacteria, maintain proper pH balance in the colon, and increase the bulk and frequency of bowel movements.

- *Kim Chee:* Fermented cabbage that has many powerful *phytochemicals* that fight cancer. The same lactic acids that help preserve the fermented cabbage also encourage intestinal health. It is fat free and cholesterol free. [93]

- *Natto:* Japanese breakfast dish. Made from soybeans fermented by natto bacillus, *natto* is a good source of protein. A fibrinolytic enzyme found in natto is *nattokinase*, which is reported to reduce and prevent blood clots.[94]

- *Sauerkraut:* Although sauerkraut—German for sour cabbage—is thought of as a German invention, Chinese laborers building the Great Wall of China over 2,000 years ago ate it as standard fare. And the Dutch used sauerkraut on their ships, as it did not need refrigeration and helped prevent scurvy.[95]

A study recently done at the University of New Mexico found a relationship between the eating of cabbage or sauerkraut and a reduced risk of breast cancer.[96]

Based on current scientific studies, and recorded history dating back thousands of years, fermented foods are a healthy addition to the diet. Check your local health food store for these products or find a cookbook that will guide you into the world of fermented foods. For several excellent fermented recipes, go to Mercola.com.

②③ Juicing For Health

Some years ago, the popular TV figure and "juice man," Jay Kordich, produced an infomercial touting the healthy benefits of freshly prepared juices. He explained how they were a good addition to an already healthy diet and a great addition to a not so healthy one. On this infomercial, many people gave inspiring testimonies of weight loss, renewed energy, relief from arthritic pain, lowered cholesterol, and more.

Jay was making known to the general public what many nutritionists, naturopaths, and natural healthcare practitioners already knew, and what scientific research had confirmed—that the nutrients found in fresh fruits and vegetables are health building, cancer curbing, and essential to life. And one way to get a healthy dose of these nutrients is to take them as fresh juice.

A HISTORICAL LOOK AT JUICING

The healthy benefits of freshly prepared juice have been touted for decades (and even further back in history). Pioneering physician Max Gerson, M.D., began using fresh juices (and soup broth) to heal his cancer patients in the 1940s. And nutrition researcher Dr. Bircher-Brenner (1867–1936) found that his green-juice preparations were among the most potent foods available. Eminent teacher Norman Walker, D.C., recovered from serious illness by eating raw foods and juicing, as he discusses in his many books.

It seems there is an ongoing debate: to juice or not to juice. Some folks say eat only the whole fruit or vegetable. Others say blend the produce in a high-speed blender and eat it all for the fiber.

I believe you can benefit from both, but in adding fresh juice and extracting the fiber, you have a highly bio-available source of vitamins and minerals. Think of it as a liquid vitamin-mineral pill.

As a note, stick mostly with juicing vegetables because fruits (and carrots too) are high in sugar. Natural sugar, yes, but a big glass of apple or grape juice will provide enough sugar to upset the glucose levels in the body. This is particularly important for anyone with blood sugar problems. If you juice fruits such as apples, grapefruit, or oranges, limit intake to only four-to-six-ounces a day.

BUT IT'S SO TIME CONSUMING!

Some people say it takes too much time to juice. Maybe! But maybe we've become a nation that doesn't want to think much about food preparation. Listen to what Eric Schlosser has to say in *Fast Food Nation:*

> Hundreds of millions of people buy fast food every day without much thought, unaware of the subtle and not so subtle ramifications of their purchases. They rarely consider where this food came from, how it was made, what it is doing to the community around them. They just grab their tray off the counter, find a table, take a seat, unwrap the contents, and dig in.
> The whole experience is transitory and soon forgotten. I've written this book out of a belief that people should know what lies behind the shiny, happy surface of every fast food transaction. They should know what really lurks between those sesame-seed buns. As the old saying goes: You are what you eat.[97]

———

KATHRYN'S JUICING STORY

"IT WAS A WOW MOMENT FOR ME!"

It was a "wow" moment for me! We were working on this manuscript, and I went by the office to talk with Ron (contributing author and Vice President of Get Healthy, America!) He was in the office kitchen preparing freshly squeezed green juice (collards, broccoli, kale, romaine, and a little carrot).

I watched as he took the five vegetables from the refrigerator, cleaned them well, cut them to a size that would fit into the juice hopper, and began the juicing process.

When the juice was prepared, he disassembled the juice machine, discarded the pulp, and washed the parts. Watching intently as he prepared his healthy beverage—having done it myself hundreds of times—I said to him, "Man, that's a lot of time and effort!"

Now here is the "wow" moment. He looked at me and replied, "No longer than making bacon and eggs, then cleaning up the greasy mess."

His comment got my attention. Every day, we spend time in the kitchen preparing something to eat. And almost for sure (unless we are simply zapping a TV dinner in the microwave), it will take as much time as making that glass of juice. So why not spend part of your kitchen time making a juice that will give your body ultimate nourishment?

NUTRIENTS GALORE IN FRESH JUICE

Raw fruits and vegetables are nature's storehouse of nutrients. From vitamins to minerals to enzymes, these foods have it all! They are also rich in phytochemicals—plant compounds that have been shown to combat cancer and other degenerative diseases.

Different phytochemicals are being discovered all the time, and it is not possible for them all to be put into a capsule. This is why it is recommended that even if you do take vitamin and mineral supplements, a wide variety of fruits and vegetables should be included in the diet every day. Juicing is a good way to ensure you've received your optimal daily amounts.

Whenever possible, buy organically grown produce free of pesticide residue. If you cannot obtain organic produce, thoroughly scrub and wash your vegetables. Generally, skins may be left on except in fruits such as oranges, grapefruit, kiwi, pineapple, and mango. Vegetable washes are readily available in most stores today. They help remove soil, dirt, and wax from the surface of fruits/vegetables.

Keep in mind that juicing is an adjunct to an already healthy diet. To make sure you are getting your daily requirement of fiber, your meal plan should also be rich in fruits and vegetables with their skins, plus, of course, high-quality protein and a variety of whole-grains.

LINDA'S JUICING STORY

"I FELT LIKE EVERYTHING BAD IN MY BODY WAS DISSOLVING"

I met Linda, a reflexologist, at the Optimum Health Institute, San Diego, CA, in 2007. (Reflexology is a science that deals with reflex points/meridians/locations in the feet, each of which is reflexively related to each and every organ in the body. Stimulating these points with massage helps to stimulate the nerves and bring blood, oxygen, and nutrients to those areas.)

I found Linda very insightful, knowledgeable about nutrition, and excellent at her job. We were talking about fresh juice one day, and I asked her to write down her remarkable story, which she shared with me during a reflexology session. Here is what she wrote:

———

"I was born with chronic bronchitis and given antibiotics three to four times a year as a child. I was raised on Southern food, which included mostly cooked, greasy foods with lots of bacon fat.

At the age of forty-four, everything in my body started to change. I began to develop osteoarthritis, my eyes were going bad, and my legs and arms were numb in the morning. I went to the eye doctor who told me this was normal "for my age" and I needed glasses. Each year, I got stronger glasses until I was forty-seven.

One day, I visited a friend who had tried to get me to drink juice for years. This time, I said yes. She gave me a straight carrot juice, which I thought was awful. Then she gave me an apple juice, which was wonderful. She said she should have mixed them so they would have tasted better at my first try.

I continued stopping by her house for a while to have the juice. Then, I noticed one day that I didn't need my glasses to read. Everything was sharp and clear without glasses. The glasses made things fuzzy. You didn't have to hit me over the head with a hammer to get my attention! I knew the juice had made a difference.

After that, a neighbor let me borrow his juicer for two weeks. I juiced fresh vegetables and fruits three times a day. I couldn't get enough. I loved it!

So I bought a juicer and started juicing. I felt like everything "bad" in my body was rinsing away. At fifty, I went back to the same eye doctor. I told him my eyes had gotten stronger, and he just laughed. Then he did the examination, which confirmed that my eyes were better. He also told me the growth in my eye was gone (I didn't even know it was there).

He asked me what I had done. I told him juicing, chiropractic, and eye exercises. He said maybe the chiropractor had helped. But he asked me two more times what it was I drank before I left his office.

Juicing changed my life. I've always juiced once a day since that time. For six years, I juiced three times a day faithfully, even carrying my juicer to work, but then fell off my routine. Now at sixty, I'm starting back juicing and can already feel the difference. Sometimes I feel so good, almost as though I don't have a body!"

WHY DID LINDA'S HEALTH IMPROVE FROM JUICING?

Linda's results were dramatic, and not everyone will receive the same rapid benefits. But hundreds of scientific studies, and all nutrition textbooks, confirm that vitamin A (which Linda was getting in carrots) is necessary to maintain good eyesight. And the other nutrients she was getting were helping with her other conditions.

Linda was also juicing plenty of dark, leafy-green vegetables, which are excellent sources of the phytochemicals lutein and zeaxanthin, known to build healthy eyes. And take note of her consistency—she made fresh vegetable juice a part of her diet every day for several years!

WHAT ABOUT CANNED & PREPARED JUICES?

Keep in mind that we are talking here about freshly prepared juices. They are far healthier than canned, bottled, or refrigerated choices. When you make them fresh and drink them immediately, or as soon as possible, you retain the most health-giving nutrients.

Pasteurized bottled or canned juices do not provide you with the same health benefits as live, freshly prepared juices. Living enzymes present only in living, raw foods are the key. Enzymes are needed for every chemical reaction that takes place in your body. No mineral, vitamin, or hormone can do its work without enzymes.

By buying the best produce available, properly preparing it for juicing, and processing it in your own juicer, you will produce the most healthful, nutrient-rich drinks possible—drinks chock-full of living enzymes, vitamins, minerals, and phytochemicals, all nutrients that will improve your health.

There are numerous juicers in the marketplace–from inexpensive types to heavy duty varieties with multiple functions. Check *www. gethealthyamerica.biz* for a variety of juicers.

ACTION PLAN FOR FRESHLY SQUEEZED JUICES
GENERAL RECOMMENDATIONS

- Buy a good juicer, and place it on the kitchen counter where it is convenient. Through the years, I have owned several juicers. I love my Champion Juicer because it also allows you to make natural ice cream, non-dairy sorbet, specialty fillings, and other unusual foods that need to be pureed.

- Keep a supply of washed and dried vegetables and fruits in plastic bags in the refrigerator (prepare them the day you shop so the whole process will be more convenient during the week). Most health food stores have specially designed plastic bags that extend the storage life of vegetables and fruits.

- Whenever possible, buy organic produce to avoid pesticides. Drink the juice as soon after making as possible. For best absorption, take juice separate from meals—an hour before or two hours after.

- Use juicing as an addition to an already healthy diet. Be sure to also eat whole foods rich in nutrients and fiber.

BODY-SPECIFIC VEGETABLES & FRUITS

Apples— Good source of malic acid, which improves cell energy; apples also contain pectin that binds cholesterol.

Beets— Considered a blood-builder, beets detoxify the liver and are rich in the B vitamin folic acid, vitamins A and C, and potassium.

Carrots— Extremely rich in vitamin A. They are good for eyes. Caution: carrots are high on the Glycemic Index, so use judiciously.

Celery— Raw celery contains vitamins A, B-complex, C, E, and minerals. Celery helps to break down the crystal deposits in joints, which cause arthritis pain.

Cucumber— High mineral content. The skin of the cucumber has the valuable cell salts and vitamins in and near it. Hence, it should not be peeled. Excellent as a diuretic (relieves water retention), and for balancing hormones.

Dark, Leafy-Green Vegetables: Good sources of many vitamins and minerals. The darker the leaves, the more nutrients in the plant.

Ginger— Known to relieve migraines, motion sickness, and inflammation, ginger gives any juice a good flavor; it is an excellent digestive aid.

Lemons— Good for kidneys and the liver as a cleanser. Add ¼ of a lemon to any juice combination.

Parsley— One of the richest food sources of most minerals. Helps reduce water retention.

Pineapple— Good as a natural digestive aid and for bones.

Watermelon — In season purchase a watermelon (choose organic whenever possible). The whole watermelon, including seeds and rind, can be juiced for bioflavonoids and chlorophyll.

Zucchini— Rich in minerals and mild tasting. It is a good source of vitamin C, low in sugar, and good for diabetics.

GET HEALTHY, AMERICA!

FRESH JUICE CLEANSES

Spring Cleansing Cocktail
  2 sprigs parsley
  ½ apple
  1 small carrot
  1 very small beet
  2 stalks celery

• Juice all ingredients. Drink immediately.

Cabbage Juice
(Powerful anti-cancer, anti-tumor benefits)
  ¼ to ½ head cabbage
  2 carrots or 1 apple

• Push ingredients through a juicer and drink immediately.

Green Drink
Use kale, dark lettuce, cilantro, parsley, Swiss chard, beet greens, or any other dark, leafy-green vegetable or herb. Juice the quantities you desire. You may add an apple, carrot, or slice of ginger to sweeten or flavor. This is an excellent anti-cancer, chlorophyll-rich drink.

②④ Powerful Protein—Key to Health

Over fifty years ago, research scientists, backed by several major cereal companies, set out to prove once and for all that mom was right when she said, "Eat your breakfast so you'll do good in school." In the Iowa Breakfast Studies, researchers W.W. Tuttle and Kate Daum showed that if a person ate one ounce of protein in the morning, their job performances at specific tasks were better than those who ate no protein at all or less than one ounce.

One area that interested the Iowa researchers was the effect of breakfast on schoolchildren. In one study of seven boys between the ages of twelve and fourteen, the researchers found that boys could not pedal as hard or as long on a bicycle when they missed breakfast.

> "It was the opinion of the school principal and of the teacher that breakfast was a material asset to the boys both in the matter of attitude and scholastic accomplishment," Tuttle and Daum wrote.[98] That was fifty years ago. Do you think today's principals and teachers would be as likely to link diet to student behavior and attitude?

Alicia never ate breakfast. For that matter, she didn't eat much of anything. And, like the schoolchildren in the 1950s, she was low on energy—almost all the time!

ALICIA BENSON'S STORY

"I'M SO TIRED IN THE AFTERNOON, I JUST FEEL LIKE GOING TO BED"

Alicia came into the clinic with her mother. She was a pretty sixteen-year old, but was extremely thin (bordering on skinny), very pale, and looked sad. As she slumped down in the office chair, she wrapped her arms around her midriff and appeared aloof, staring down at her feet. During most of our meeting, Alicia rocked back and forth gently, with her arms wrapped tightly around her midriff. She had very little eye contact with me, and none at all with her mother.

Mrs. Benson had scheduled the appointment to see Dr. Wright a few months prior. Alicia reluctantly agreed to come in for a complete physical. They were in my office to talk about Alicia's diet. Mom did most of the talking, and after a little "chit-chat," we got down to business. I looked directly at Alicia.

"Alicia, you are very thin. And you don't look like you feel well."

She squirmed a little in her chair. "I'm ok. It's just that sometimes I get tired in the afternoon and just feel like going to bed."

"Well, how can I help you?"

"My mom wanted me to come. She says I don't eat right."

Mrs. Benson interrupted. "Well, she doesn't. I can't get her to eat hardly anything. I'm worried."

Alicia rolled her eyes.

"Let's talk about what you eat. Tell me about breakfast."

"Oh, no breakfast! I can't stand the way it makes me feel. I'd rather do without."

"Okay. Then lunch. What about lunch?" I queried.

"We get to leave the campus for lunch, and there are a couple of fast-food restaurants across the street. We go there."

"And what do you eat?"

"Well, my friends order meals, and I eat some of their fries. And a coke. I don't eat the hamburger because I don't eat meat."

As a nutritionist, I knew that a fast-food burger wasn't the healthiest choice on the planet, but I was hoping she ate one just to get some protein.

I said, "Well, what about dinner?"

"Well, Mom always makes a full meal with meat, potatoes, and vegetables, but I don't usually eat it. I don't eat meat, and I don't like vegetables. I sometimes just make instant noodles and go to bed."

Mrs. Benton kept looking at me frantically, as if to beg me to do something. I had to think a minute about where to start with Alicia. There had been no diagnosis of anorexia from the doctor.

"Alicia, I see that Dr. Wright is ordering some laboratory testing. That will tell us if you have any more serious problems. But regardless of the tests, I think you're probably not eating enough food, and for sure you are low on protein."

I told Alicia about the Iowa Breakfast Studies and how the boys who didn't get enough protein weren't really sick; they just weren't performing the best they could. We talked about how her blood sugar was erratic, rising and plummeting throughout the day as a result of her diet.

"You probably feel better after the French fries or the noodles. And I'm sure the coke gives you a lift as your blood sugar goes up. But then, you get tired when it comes racing down. Right?"

"Well, I don't know about that blood sugar stuff, but I am so tired a lot."

I asked her to start eating protein—just an ounce or two for breakfast. Since she didn't eat meat but said she liked eggs and cheese, I suggested a hard-boiled egg or a piece of cheese in the morning before school, or maybe cottage cheese and raw nuts.

After I insisted that she also have some form of protein for lunch and dinner, we went into more detail about her terrible diet. She needed fresh fruits, vegetables, and whole-grains—basically a well-balanced diet. She weighed one hundred ten pounds, so we calculated that she needed about forty grams of protein a day.

As they got up to leave my office, I said, "One more thing. Do you want to have a family one day?"

"Oh, yes! Very much!"

"Well then, let me tell you something really important. The food choices you are making today are influencing your growth and development in these critical teenage years. But your choices today will also have long-term effects, Alicia. I would hate to see you jeopardize your ability to get pregnant in the future, so be sure to work on the diet changes we've talked about."

"Okay. I will."

———

I have thought about Alicia through the years. By now, she is a woman of childbearing years. I hope that she made the necessary dietary changes we talked about, is happily married, and has a healthy brood of children—and that she is feeding them well!

PROTEIN'S IMPORTANT JOBS

Most people think of protein as the T-bone steak on their plate, the eggs that hold their omelet together, or the chicken breast inside a fast-food sandwich. And they are right. Protein is generally the food we build a meal around. But many other foods besides meat or eggs contain protein. Vegetable sources include tofu and other soy products, nuts, seeds, and legumes.

Whatever your personal dietary selections, your muscles, organs, and immune system are made up mostly of protein and will use it to maintain health. The protein you eat will form specialized protein molecules that have very specific jobs. Whether you're running, sleeping, watching the TV, fighting off an infection, or building cardiac muscle, protein is doing important work in your body.

AMINO ACIDS–THE MOLECULES OF PROTEIN

When you eat foods that contain protein, the digestive juices in your stomach and intestines break it down into basic units called *amino acids*. These amino acids are then used to make the proteins your body needs to maintain muscles, bones, blood, and body organs. Proteins are sometimes described as looking like "long strings of differently shaped pearls." Each of these pearls is an amino acid. The amino acids can join together to make thousands of different proteins.

Now here is the important point you should know about protein: Your body cannot make ten of these amino acids, so you must get them from eating protein-rich foods. These ten are called *essential amino acids* because it's essential that you get them from the foods you eat. They are arginine (required for the young, but not for adults), histidine, isoleucine, leucine, lysine, methionine, phenylalanine, threonine, tryptophan, and valine.

DIFFERENT KINDS OF PROTEIN

Protein is found in animal sources like meat, fish, eggs, and milk. It is also present in vegetables such as beans, grains, nuts, and legumes.

If you are vegetarian or vegan and want to make absolutely sure you are getting adequate protein, you can combine any lentil with any grain. For instance, the following foods would be good choices for entrees: bean burritos, bean soup with brown rice, or corn tortillas and beans.

JASON'S STORY

"I BECAME A VEGETARIAN BECAUSE OF MY GIRLFRIEND, BUT I DON'T FEEL GOOD"

Jason worked as a laboratory aid at the Tahoma Clinic. I didn't know him well, but had seen him around dozens of times. One rainy, winter afternoon, he came around the corner to the clinic to talk with the head nurse, Sandy. I was standing at her desk, so became involved in the conversation.

"Something is wrong. I don't feel well. I thought you could help."

As it always is with a nutritional approach to health, the answer is never as simple as, "Take this, and call me in the morning."

Sandy put her pen down and asked him to describe how he felt. It was obvious from looking at him that he felt bad. His color was horrible—almost gray.

"I am weak and tired a lot. My girlfriend says I've been depressed and moody lately."

The conversation went on at length and finally, being the nutritionist, I asked him about his diet.

"Well, my girlfriend is a vegetarian, so I decided to become one. I haven't had any meat or eggs for eight months."

I asked him more questions about that. "What do you eat for protein? Are you sure you are getting enough?"

"I never think about that. I just eat until I am full."

Of course, the next question was, "What do you eat?" And not surprisingly, he rattled off a whole array of foods—all nutrient-devoid—that were his standard fare.

"I eat lots of instant noodles, the kind that cook in five minutes. I like sweets, of course. And candy. I eat lots of bread (white) and margarine to fill me up. Sometimes my girlfriend and I make rice (white) and beans. Sometimes we go out for Mexican food, no cheese of course. Sometimes we eat soy burgers."

Sandy and I had both worked with hundreds of Tahoma Clinic patients, some vegetarian, some not. We had seen eating habits of every sort (one man recorded that his breakfast consisted of marsh-mallows and beer).

I knew that vegetarianism vs. non-vegetarianism could be a touchy subject, especially for diehard vegetarians. But I also knew that veg-etarianism was not the right choice for everyone. I'd had numerous people tell me over the years that they "just felt better when they ate a little meat." As a clinician, my job was to help them attain their best health through the most appropriate diet for them. Sometimes that was vegetarian. Sometimes it was not.

Sandy and I made eye contact. It was Sandy who made the first suggestion (a vegetarian herself). "Would it be acceptable to you to try eating a little fish? Say a little salmon? It could be that you need more protein."

He did not object at all; in fact, he seemed relieved. "I could try some fish."

The conversation ended, and Jason went on his way.

A couple of weeks later, Jason stopped in to tell Sandy that he was feeling much better. Neither Sandy nor I were surprised. We were just happy that this handsome young man, generally full of energy and vigor, was back on a nutritional path that, for him, provided what his body needed to function at its peak.

———

The eminent Roger Williams, M.D., in 1956, was the first to rec-ognize that humans differ biochemically from each other. He wrote that while we all have the same physical and metabolic processes, we are each very different. He also said that what is taking place in one individual's body may be quite different than the reactions in another of the same age, sex. and size.[99]

His observations led Dr. Williams to theorize that each individual also had unique nutritional needs, and that determining and meeting those needs would help combat disease.

And so the story goes with protein, as with all nutritional requirements. Making sure that you are getting the appropriate kinds and amount as outlined above is simply one more key in helping you reach optimum health.

ACTION PLAN
GENERAL RECOMMENDATIONS FOR DIETARY PROTEIN INTAKE

- Eat a balanced diet that includes plenty of fresh vegetables, fruits, and grains. Eat a protein source—vegetarian or not—as an adjunct to the above foods. To figure your daily protein requirements, a general rule of thumb for adults is .9 grams per kilogram of body weight. A kilogram is 2.2 pounds. Thus, a 60-kilogram (132-pound) woman probably needs about 54 grams of protein a day.[100]

- For those who do not think in terms of grams, here is a good visual example from one of my very old textbooks:

A kilogram (kg) equals 2.2 pounds (which can be visualized, roughly, by thinking of slightly more than 2 pounds of butter or margarine, or flour or sugar, or a quart of milk). A pencil eraser or one lima bean weighs about 1 gram (gm); a penny weighs nearly 3 gm; and a shelled egg about 50 gm.[101]

DIETARY TIPS

- Beef is difficult to digest (think of how much chewing it requires). Choose beef sparingly.

- Choose meat protein only three times a week instead of daily.

- Choose wild salmon over farmed varieties because it is higher in nutrition.

- If you are vegetarian, make sure you understand the principles of food-combining and protein intake.

- Meat eaters should try to find organic sources of meat to avoid chemicals, hormones, and other toxins.

- No matter what your dietary choices, make the biggest share of your meals from vegetables, followed by fruits and whole-grain foods.

- Try new ideas occasionally, like a vegetarian sandwich, home-made vegetable soup with whole-grain muffins, bean burritos with brown rice, or soy burgers.

2️5 Sprout for Health

> Wanted: A live vegetable that will grow in any climate, rivals meat in nutritional value and tomatoes in vitamin C, matures in two to five days, may be planted any day of the year, requires neither soil nor sunshine, has no waste, and is tastiest eaten raw. [102]

This was a puzzling ad written by Dr. Clive McCag of Cornell University in the early 1970s. It would have perplexed the world had it been printed in the newspapers of that time. Today, some thirty years later, many vegetarians and people interested in a special kind of natural nutrition know what type of vegetable Dr. McCag was describing—sprouts!

SPROUTS—THE NEW & TRENDY FOOD

Considered novel and trendy, fresh sprouts are an essential of the new avant-garde eating craze—raw foods! Actually, eating raw foods and the sprouting of grains and seeds is as old as writing. Recorded history tells us that sprouts were eaten by such ancient civilizations as the Egyptians, the Chinese, the East Indians, and the Hebrews of the Old Testament. Now, contemporary scientists are studying sprouts for their health benefits. [103]

Dr. Paul Talalay at John Hopkins School of Medicine and his colleagues isolated a phytochemical called of *sulforaphane* found in broccoli. They published their findings in the Proceedings of the National Academy of Sciences, and were credited with a major breakthrough in understanding the potential link between cruciferous vegetable consumption and reduced cancer risk. [104]

And studies from Tokyo University of Agriculture and the Japan Institute for the Control of Aging revealed that individuals who ate 3½-ounces of broccoli sprouts daily for just one week reduced their overall cholesterol level and increased their levels of HDL or good cholesterol.[105]

ALL SPROUTS ARE EXCELLENT IN FOOD VALUE

But don't stop with broccoli sprouts! All sprouts are unequaled in nutritional value. Rich in B-vitamins, protein, and amino acids, they increase in their nutritional value during the fast-growing period dramatically over the original hard grain.

Sprouts are very easy to grow—right in your own kitchen. You can buy all sorts of sprouting containers and books about sprouting at a natural food store.

You will see a tiny white protrusion when the plant has begun to visibly grow. When the protrusion is approximately the length of the grain or seed, it is ready to eat.

Sprouts, all kinds of them (seeds, legumes, grains), combine well with all other natural foods whether they are fruits, nuts, vegetables, or roots. Calorie for calorie and nutrient for nutrient, they are an excellent source of nutrition, very inexpensive, and a good addition to any diet.

26 Wheatgrass—Nature's Most Potent Drink

Wheatgrass juice was popularized by the late Ann Wigmore, founder of the Hippocrates Health Institute, which opened its doors in 1958 in Boston. The Institute's program consisted of consuming living, raw foods—sprouts, seeds, raw fruits, and vegetables—and several ounces of wheatgrass juice every day.

Since that time, alternative health practitioners have preached the benefits of wheatgrass, due largely to its chlorophyll content. Chlorophyll is the pigment that gives plants their green color. It absorbs sunlight necessary for photosynthesis, hence the term "liquid sunshine." Wheatgrass is also a rich source of vitamins, minerals, and trace elements.

Dr. Ann's work at the Hippocrates Institute has produced numerous testimonies of guests who claim cures of practically every known ailment—high blood pressure, diabetes, obesity, gastritis, stomach ulcers, pancreas and liver troubles, asthma, glaucoma, eczema, skin problems, constipation, hemorrhoids, diverticulosis, fatigue, female problems, arthritis, athlete's foot, and cancer.

Since wheatgrass juice is mostly chlorophyll, many call it the blood of the plant. It is very similar in structure to human blood. "In experiments on anemic animals, blood counts returned to normal after four to five days of receiving chlorophyll." [106]

THE ANN WIGMORE WHEATGRASS STORY

"INSTINCT-GUIDED CREATURES LEFT TO THEMSELVES DO NOT MAKE MISTAKES"

Ann Wigmore was a Lithuanian born in 1910. She lived with her naturalist grandmother who taught her of the healing power of herbs. At age sixteen, Ann came to America, and shortly after was in a car accident that broke both legs. Her doctors wanted to amputate in order to save her life, but she refused.

At home, she was shunned by mother and father who wanted her to comply with the doctor's orders to amputate. She spent her days in a backyard lawn chair nibbling on grass. She watched the greenish-blue ring—gangrene—as it grew bigger on her legs.

One day, her puppy who had not come near her for months, began to lick her legs for the first time, and she knew she would recover. Her doctors informed her family that she was out of danger. She remembered her Grandmother's saying, "Instinct-guided creatures left to themselves do not make mistakes."

Ann Wigmore healed completely, and X-rays showed that the bones had knitted together very well. Amazingly enough, her legs became so strong that she later ran in the Boston Marathon. She attributed much of her healing to the chlorophyll-rich grass she chewed all summer.[107]

THE OPTIMUM HEALTH INSTITUTE— RAW FOOD & WHEATGRASS

I've had the good fortune to visit the Optimum Health Institute (OHI) in Lemon Grove, California, numerous times. Contributing author, Ron Lowrie has also been a guest.

An oasis nestled in an urban environment and surrounded by

organic, lush gardens, one can go to OHI to rest, recover, pray, learn, and enjoy some of the healthiest foods on the planet.

The program includes raw, living, organic vegetarian foods and juice fasting. It also incorporates colon cleansing, lymphatic exercises, and wheatgrass therapy. At the end of a stay at OHI, participants gather to share how their stay has transformed their lives.

Easy-to-reach, and reasonably priced, OHI is a great place to visit! www.optimumhealth.org.

EDIE MAE'S CANCER STORY

In 1973, Edie Mae discovered that she had breast cancer. After a long and grueling period involving doctor visits, recommendations of chemotherapy, radiation, and the like, Edie Mae chose instead to pursue healing through the use of living foods. In *How I Conquered Cancer Naturally*, she talks about her experience with the Hippocrates Institute, wheatgrass, and *abscisic acid*, a natural ingredient found in the drink. This book is out of print, but worth searching for on the internet. About abscisic acid, she writes:

> Believe me, we had to do some mind-stretching when we started considering the idea of drinking wheatgrass and eating only live, raw foods to bring about a reversal with my malignant breast cancer. Now we were very grateful to be in a position where we could begin to understand it from the scientific viewpoint.
>
> Within the next year, the doctor's research uncovered the unknown ingredient that could reverse the growth of a cancerous tumor. Our doctor made it known to us that it is the abscisic acid in the wheatgrass that reverses the growth, and in the experimental tests, abscisic acid in its natural form was found to be deadly against any form of cancer...and it only took a very small amount of the abscisic acid. When some live tumor-bearing animals were given

injections of abscisic acid, their tumors quickly deteriorated. As I understand it, this work is still in the research stages ...[108]

WHERE TO BUY WHEATGRASS

Wheatgrass is available in natural food stores, and I have even seen it in many grocery stores. It is sold in trays of various sizes. You can also grow it yourself; many books are available with instructions.

To make wheatgrass, you clip the grass at the root level when it is four-to-five-inches tall. These grass blades are then put through a special wheatgrass juicer. Most standard juicers are not designed to extract the chlorophyll from the grass.

2 7 Where Did All the Whole Grains Go?

I never knew what a grain of whole-wheat looked like until I was thirty years old. I had only seen packaged loaves of bread, bags of white flour, boxes of cream of wheat, and numerous baked goods, mostly homemade with white flour. Actually, I'd never really thought about it until I began to study nutrition. Then I read Dr. David Reuben's book, *The Save Your Life Diet*. It changed the way I looked at refined foods (foods that have been stripped of nutrition by the modern refining process). It also helped me understand the importance of eating whole grains. While the book is out of print, you may find it on the internet.

THE GOODNESS OF WHOLE-WHEAT

Whole-wheat kernels are a rich source of nutrition. Inside each tiny seed are three parts—the endosperm, the bran, and the germ. Keep in mind that when you eat whole-wheat products, you are eating all three, as described below:

- Endosperm: What most of us are familiar with is the endosperm—the starch, gluten, or white flour that we eat in most of our foods. This includes pies, breads, cookies, crackers, etc.

- Bran: The wheat bran is the outer coat of the kernel, similar to what you see when you pop corn. A good source of fiber, it is also rich in protein and B-vitamins. When whole-wheat grain is processed into white flour, the fiber is removed.

- Wheat Germ: The wheat germ is the sprouting section of the wheat kernel and is rich in B-vitamins, wheat-germ oil, and trace minerals.

NUTRIENT-POOR WHITE FLOUR

By the time the whole-wheat kernel has been whittled down to white flour, almost all of the nutrients are gone. Between 70 and 85% of the vitamin and mineral content is removed when whole wheat is refined into white flour. These lost nutrients are critical to good health, as you will read below.

- B-6: Involved in more body functions than almost any other nutrient.

- Magnesium: Deficiency causes heart problems and constipation.

- Manganese: Needed for healthy nerves and immune system.

- Fiber: Protective against colon cancer.

- Zinc: Important for prostate gland and reproductive organs.

- Potassium: Critical for a regular heartbeat.

- Copper: Early deficiency sign is osteoporosis.

- Pantothenic acid: Involved with nerve health.

- Folic acid: Nutrient protective against birth defects.

- Protein: Important for growth and repair.

VITAMIN E & WHOLE-WHEAT

Vitamin E is the body's naturally occurring lubricant or anti-clotting agent as well as a very powerful antioxidant that helps destroy harmful free radicals (toxins) in the body. Without adequate amounts of vitamin E the risk of heart disease, cancer, and many other degenerative diseases increases drastically.

> Around the year 1900, the average American ate at least 100 I.U. (international units) of natural vitamin E each day in their food. The primary source was stone-ground whole-wheat bread. In the late 1800s, the rolling mill was invented, and this machine separated the wheat germ from the wheat bran, leaving only the kernel. White bread was born, and it became very popular. However, this milling process removed many of the vital nutrients essential to our bodies, including the majority of the vitamin E, as the wheat germ and wheat bran contained these nutrients.[109]

Because stone ground wheat can become rancid very quickly, the simple process of removing the wheat germ and wheat bran allows the product to be kept for indefinite periods of time. This made the product much easier to store and sell, but it also robbed the body of some very essential nutrients.

> Vitamin E has also been taken out of grocery store variety processed foods because the vitamin E will cause the food to turn rancid much more quickly, which diminishes the shelf life of the products. Vitamin E is the only substance that is not added back into most foods as this creates a significant problem in the distribution and shelf life of these products.[110]

2 8 The Power of Whole Foods

Thousands upon thousands of well-documented scientific studies recorded in prestigious medical journals from around the world confirm that whole foods have the extraordinary power to heal the human body. From annoying conditions such as headaches and PMS to asthma or urinary-tract infections, nature has a remedy that can ease, improve, or even eradicate the condition.

What's more, whole foods have powerful positive influences on the grim "killer diseases" of the twenty-first century such as heart disease, diabetes, and cancer. The possibilities and power of whole foods are endless, and included here are just a small sampling of their health-giving and healing benefits. By all means, don't stop researching what foods might benefit you. Who knows—you might find lurking inside your kitchen cupboard a food that will help you eat your way out of a dilemma!

FOODS WITH ANTI-CANCER PROPERTIES

Figs have long been talked about for their anticancer properties. Figs contain an ingredient called *benzaldehyde* that has been shown to shrink tumors in humans, according to Japanese studies.

A study by Dr. Michael Wargovich, M.D., found that mice eating *garlic* had 75% fewer colon tumors.[111]

Dr. Helmut Sies of Germany, found that lycopene is twice as powerful as beta-carotene at "quenching singlet oxygen," a toxic molecule that can trigger cancer. *Tomatoes* are the best source of lycopene. [112]

Grapefruit juice is also an anticancer food. A study has found that smokers who drank six ounces of grapefruit juice three times a day boosted their levels of an anticancer compound in their urine.[113]

Watercress (eaten frequently) can significantly reduce the precursor to cancer (DNA damage to blood cells). A study showed that, in addition to reducing this damage, it also increased the resistance of those cells to further damage caused by free radicals.[114]

FOODS WITH BRAIN-BENEFITING COMPOUNDS

Green tea possesses EGCG (epigallocatechin gallate), with anticancer properties and brain cell protection. Steep green tea for at least five minutes to receive the benefits; instant, bottled, or herb teas lack the antioxidants necessary for the benefits.[115]

Selenium (found in Brazil nuts) eases depression. In one study, people with low selenium levels were more depressed and tired. Studies showed that once they ate foods containing selenium, they felt better. Selenium is also in tuna, swordfish, and sunflower seeds.[116]

A recent study found that *zinc* improved the memory of seventh-graders who were given 20-milligrams of zinc a day. They performed better in recalling information than students who were given 10-milligrams or students given a placebo with no zinc.[117] Zinc rich foods include beef, sesame seeds, pumpkin seeds, and crimini mushrooms.

FOODS FOR ULCERS & STOMACH-RELATED PROBLEMS

Garnett Cheney, M.D., conducted a study in the 1950s showing that a quart of fresh *cabbage* juice every day relieved ulcer pain and healed duodenal and gastric ulcers even better than traditional drugs.[118]

Studies have proved that only ½ teaspoon of ground ginger can eliminate or reduce seasickness. [119]

FOODS WITH HEART & ARTERY BENEFITS

Antioxidants contained in pomegranate juice may help reduce the formation of fatty deposits on artery walls. Antioxidants are compounds
that limit cell damage. Scientists tested the juice and found that it
combats hardening of the arteries and related diseases, such as heart
attacks and strokes. Claudio Napoli, a professor of medicine in Italy,
states, "In this experimental study, we have established that *polyphe-
nols* [antioxidant chemicals] and other natural compounds contained
in the pomegranate juice may retard atherogenesis."[120]

Raspberries are high in natural aspirin—*salicylic acid*—and thought
to inhibit atherosclerosis, which suggests the possibility that salicylic
acid consumed in foods may provide a similar benefit. A 100-gram
serving (about 3/4 a cup) of red raspberries contains around 5-mil-
ligrams of salicylic acid.[121]

One of civilization's oldest medicines—*raw onions*—are exceptionally
strong antioxidants. A rich source of dietary *quercetin*, all kinds of
onions are thought to thin blood, lower cholesterol, and help keep
arteries clean and open.[122]

In a study from Loma Linda University on 31,208 Seventh-Day
Adventists, *nuts* stood out as the number one food eaten by those
who did not suffer heart attacks. Eating nuts five times a week cut
heart attack risks by half.[123]

Charles R. Dorso, M.D., of the Cornell University Medical College,
discovered after eating a large quantity of *ginger and grapefruit mar-
malade* that his blood did not coagulate as usual. He did a test by

mixing some ground ginger with his own blood platelets and found them less sticky. Dr. Dorso says the active ingredient is gingerol, a constituent of ginger that resembles aspirin.[124]

FOODS FOR FEEDING & HEALING THE EYES

An ancient herbal formula called *hachimijiogan* has long been touted to prevent the progression of cataracts. Now research finds that the remedy actually increases levels of the antioxidant *glutathione*. An excellent source of glutathione is asparagus. It is also in avocado, watermelon, oranges, and walnuts.[125]

The carotenoid *lutein* is reported to be good for eye health. Foods high in lutein are carrots, corn, red peppers, tomatoes, and dark and leafy-green vegetables. "In a study of 480 people, researchers found clearer neck (carotid) arteries in those with higher blood lutein levels."[126]

FOODS FOR LUNGS & RESPIRATORY SYSTEM

A study of Welsh men indicated that people who ate at least five *apples* per week experienced better lung function and had a lower risk for respiratory disease. Scientists believe antioxidants found in apples may ward off disease by countering oxygen's damaging effects on the lungs.[127]

Men are less likely to develop chronic lung disease if they follow a diet that closely resembles the *Mediterranean diet*, which is rich in fiber, tomatoes, olive oil, fruits, vegetables, and fish. Olive oil has a beneficial effect on cardiovascular disease by lowering cholesterol levels in the blood.

CYCLES OF LIFE

2 9 Children's Health

ABOUT DR. ELLOUISE CARROLL

Can you imagine a daycare where the children grow their own vegetables and then put their hands in the soil to harvest carrots and spinach? Where they flake their own oats to make the morning oatmeal? Where their bread is made with fresh whole wheat, ground right on site?

And where all their snacks and meals are nutritious, whole foods made to taste delicious—many times by the children themselves? Well, meet Ellouise Carroll, PhD, past director and principal of the only vegetarian preschool, childcare, and state-approved elementary school in Pierce County, Washington.

While most children in other facilities were dining on sugar-coated doughnuts, orange-flavored beverages, and packaged macaroni meals, her children were eating nutritious whole foods and discovering that they taste good! And they were learning, too, why their growing bodies needed the nutrition that only whole foods can provide.

Dr. Ellouise was the principal at ECE (Early Childhood Education) Academy for over twenty years. ECE Academy was a trilingual school (English, Spanish, and Sign Language), where the students learned math and reading and much more with organic-growing methods.

As the Director of Childhood Education for Get Healthy, America!, she has graciously contributed this article about children and nutrition. Read every word from start to finish, as there is a wealth of information.

As you read, you will discover that she is a vegetarian and is happy to share her ideas and knowledge with us. Whether you are vegetarian or not, you will find valuable nuggets in this article that will help you raise the healthiest children possible!

FEEDING THE NEXT GENERATION
ELLOUISE CARROLL, PhD

"And God said, See I have given you every plant yielding seed that is on the face of all the land and every tree with seed in its fruit; you shall have them for food..."

Genesis 1:29 (Amplified Bible)

Let's put this into perspective. What's the most important thing you can do for your children? Eating correctly is not the right answer. Helping them into the saving knowledge of Jesus Christ is the right answer.

But after that, you can make an incredible difference in your children's lives by helping them make healthy lifestyle choices. So, how do you do that?

First, let me tell you a little about myself. For over twenty years, I was the Director and Principal of the only vegetarian preschool, childcare, and state-approved elementary school in Pierce County, Washington.

We became vegetarian after I wrote my Master's thesis, *"Serving Healthy Foods in a Childcare."* When I began the thesis, I had a teensy goal: I just wanted to serve the children something better than sugary cereal! In my quest for more information about children, their eating habits, and what portent of the future those habits invite, I read over

300 books. What I found has affected my entire life and that of those around me.

Have you noticed that there seem to be more children with diagnosable conditions now than there were fifty years ago? Were you aware that grading systems have been revised downward in most institutions of learning? Have you noticed that there seem to be more children with obesity problems now than there were even twenty years ago?

Are you aware that the way Americans eat has drastically changed since WWII when industrialization and modern farming techniques took hold? And that since then, many types of pesticides and preservatives have been developed?

If you have answered yes to any or all of these questions, you are aware that we have a problem on our hands! It is a huge problem with no easy answers. However, if we begin to ask just twelve questions, perhaps we and our children can live healthier lives. You have heard of "12 Step Programs," so let us think of this as a Twelve Question Program!

TWELVE QUESTIONS POINTING US TOWARD HEALTH

1. What has changed since WWII regarding food production?

2. Are there really more ADHD and neurological disorders, or is it just that detection methods have improved dramatically in the last fifty years?

3. Is sugar the cause or does it just contribute to ADHD?

4. What about additives? Do they affect learning?

5. Why is it even important for me to make changes in my children's diet?

6. What health habits don't directly affect learning but are part of a healthy lifestyle?

7. What foods should I leave out for my children to be healthier?

8. Where do I start when I buy healthier foods?

9. Should I look into organic foods and, if so, why?

10. Which is better? Simple, raw, organic foods or processed, cooked foods?

11. How can I make our life and environment healthier?

12. How can I encourage my children to see a "cause and effect" between what they eat and their future health?

1. WHAT HAS CHANGED SINCE WWII REGARDING FOOD PRODUCTION?

> "Men dig their graves with their own teeth and die more by those fated instruments than the weapons of their enemies."
>
> Thomas Moffet

In discussing eating, people make all kinds of statements to justify what they eat. For instance, some will state, "Well, we've always eaten this way. What's the problem?"

The truth is that we have not always eaten this way. In fact, until after World War II, when a new, more developed level of industrialization took place, Americans ate very differently.

Writes *Diet for a Strong Heart* author Michio Kushi,

> Whole cereal grains, including brown rice, whole wheat, barley, millet, oats, rye, and corn were the cornerstone of all civilizations previous to our own. Supplemented with fresh garden vegetables,

beans, sea vegetables, fermented foods, and small amounts of seasonal fruit; seeds, nuts, and grains were eaten daily and formed the center of every meal. Animal food was consumed very sparingly and eaten with substantial quantities of grain and vegetables. Until modern times, when this way of eating changed, heart disease, cancer, and other degenerative illnesses were almost unknown.[128]

Before World War II, most foods were either home grown or grown on small farms and trucked to local markets. With no preservatives and no refrigerators, the foods were, necessarily, very fresh or they weren't eaten. Many foods were picked and then eaten within a very short period of time. Meat consumption was mostly limited to a roast on Sunday and the occasional chicken that no longer produced eggs.

After World War II, though, modern production methods and various inventions made it possible to present more food to more people, with less spoilage and, therefore, more profit. As just one small example of this change, consider wheat.

There are four parts to wheat. White flour is created by removing both the protective cover called the bran (the exterior) and the germ of the wheat. As shown by Sheryl and Mel London:

Aside from being rich in vitamins and minerals, it [bran] is the prime source of soluble fiber. Under the bran is the germ, or the embryo of the seed. When we sprout grains, this is the part that grows, and it's very rich in enzymes, protein, minerals, fat and vitamins. If we polish away both the bran and the germ, we refine the grain to the next layer, the starchy center called the endosperm. Basically, this layer gives us only carbohydrates, as in white flour.[129]

Removing the bran also removes the fiber; and it is the fiber which helps keep the intestinal system healthy.

By removing the germ of the wheat, which spoiled quickly, processed-wheat products lasted longer on the grocery shelves. No longer was it necessary to grind the wheat each day; the bread or other wheat products could be put into trucks, take quite a bit of time getting to the stores, and then take even more time sitting on the shelves. No longer was it necessary to make everything fresh at home; now it was right there on the grocery shelf, conveniently ready to buy.

Unfortunately, the processing that allows manufacturers to extend shelf life also eliminates most of the nutritional value. It is processed right out of those foods. Wheat is only one example of processing which affects our health. Most of those processes increase profits for the manufacturers and decrease the benefits to our bodies. This is the reason that we have abundant food but a lack of nutrition.

It is sometimes hard to tell that the foods we are eating are different from those in the past. After all, a potato is a potato and a loaf of bread is a loaf of bread, right? Actually, "Foods that may look familiar have, in fact, been completely reformulated. What we eat has changed more in the last forty years than in the previous forty thousand."[130]

Perhaps it's time to stop depending on the corporations, who benefit from our ignorance, and the chemists, paid by those corporations, for our nutritional information. Maybe we should go back to our organic farmers and local farmer's markets. Unfortunately, most people are not thinking about these issues nor any other issues along this line.

Hundreds of millions of people buy fast food every day without much thought, unaware of the subtle and not so subtle ramifications of their purchases. They rarely consider where this food came from, how it was made, or what it is doing to the community around them. They just grab their tray off the counter, find a table, take a seat, unwrap the paper, and dig in. The whole experience is transitory and soon forgotten. I've written this book out of a belief that people should know what lies behind the shiny, happy surface of every fast food transaction. They should know what really lurks between those sesame-seed buns. As the old saying goes: You are what you eat.[131]

And we in America are eating fake foods and "Franken foods" with alarming regularity. I define Franken foods as those foods so altered—either GMO (genetically modified), chemicalized, or in some way radically changed from what God created for people's consumption—that our bodies do not even recognize them as foods.

2. ARE THERE REALLY MORE ADHD AND NEUROLOGICAL DISORDERS, OR IS IT JUST THAT DETECTION METHODS HAVE IMPROVED DRAMATICALLY IN THE LAST FIFTY YEARS?

"It is my view that the vegetarian manner of living, by its purely physical effect on the human temperament, would most beneficially influence the lot of mankind."

Albert Einstein

Admittedly, detection methods have improved, as have treatments. But most people who have been in the Early Childhood Education (ECE) field for a length of time, as I have, will agree with me in saying that there are a larger percentage of children with problems now than when we started.

Although some much younger teachers will say that the older teachers are just getting older and are less able to tolerate children's misbehavior, this is not reality. There *are* more children with problems! Detection is great and early intervention is great, but the fact is that there are more children who need that detection and early intervention now than when I began in the ECE field in the early 1960s.

Why is this? There are many theories; following you will see some of mine.

Teen girls are focused on being model slim and deprive their bodies of many nutrients, including good fats. When these young women become pregnant, they lack the "cause and effect" mentality to see that what they eat affects their unborn child. They share this characteristic with most Americans today. The children are then born with more neurological issues. As seen from the following quote, this can have disastrous effects on the children.

> Recently, we have become aware that certain types of fats play a vital role in the formation of a baby's brain, and that when these fats are missing from the mother's diet, the baby may later suffer learning difficulties and behavioral problems. One of the most important of these fats is called docosohexiaonic acid or DHA. This fat plays an important role in the formation of the synaptic connections within the brain. These connections allow the various parts of the brain to communicate with each other and communicate with the body as well.
>
> Several recent studies, conducted in both animals and humans, have shown that babies who receive adequate amounts of this vital fat have better functioning brains and higher IQs. Those with low amounts of DHA demonstrate learning difficulties and visual problems. For the unborn baby, the source of this important fat is from the mother's blood, transferred by the placenta. After birth, it must be supplied from the mother's breast milk. Commercial formulas contain no DHA at all. Not surprisingly, several studies have shown that breast fed babies have better brain function and visual acuity than formula-fed babies.[132]

Once the mothers have the children, they feed them non-foods and Franken foods without understanding how this affects the health and mental capabilities of their children both now and in the future. As mentioned, processed foods have most of the nutrition processed out of them.

Thus, the children are in the position of the rats in one study that ate boxes instead of the food given to them; the food had been so stripped that the cardboard boxes had more nutrition than the food. Eating cardboard boxes is not acceptable for children, however, so those children don't even get that "nutrition."

These same processed foods and bad fats make up close to 100% of many children's diets. Many of these processed foods have hydrogenated oils or transfats, which then clog up the arteries. Besides the obvious problem of clogged arteries at the age of three (which has been documented), these oils do not feed the body, thus depriving it of important nutrients by taking up space in the young body.

The brain works by using the nutrients supplied by the food we eat. If there are no nutrients, it makes sense that the brain is being systematically starved. The children are filling up with processed foods instead of fresh fruits and vegetables; we think everything is fine because they are full. But their bodies are not getting nourished and neither are their brains.

Many teenage girls and boys are also on junk-food diets high in "bad fats." These fats include corn oil, sunflower oil, safflower oil, peanut oil and to a lesser degree canola oil. These oils share several unwelcome characteristics. They increase inflammation, depress the immune system and impair enzymes necessary to convert other oils (linolenic fats) into DHA oils. This results in a severe depletion of "good fats," which include fish oils and flaxseed oil. Fish oils are composed of two types of fats, EPA and DHA, both of which play a role in protecting the baby's brain from injury.[133]

Unhealthy fad diets, supported by million-dollar ad campaigns, promise to get the weight down while allowing the person to eat huge amounts of unhealthy foods. These diets appeal to people because they allow people to eat the way their taste buds have been trained to eat. The end results, though, are people with liver problems, kidney problems, heart attacks, and more.

And, sugar is found in absolutely everything, from catsup to spaghetti sauce to everything else—which brings us to the next of the twelve questions.

3. IS SUGAR THE CAUSE, OR DOES IT JUST CONTRIBUTE TO ADHD?

"Let thy food be thy medicine, and medicine thy food."

Hippocrates

Who knows? But does it matter? Sugar is detrimental to your children's mental capabilities, their physical growth, and their health. As such, it should be limited or eliminated.

Despite the recent study (sponsored by a sugar company) that said that sugar had no effect on children's behavior (they didn't even test for mental effects), most can see the effects of sugar on children. Unfortunately, this study was just slightly flawed: the "non-sugar" and "sugar" cereals were: Sugar cereal as opposed to sugar cereal with more sugar on top. Since there is so much sugar in the sugar cereal to begin with, it is not logical to say that the sugar added onto a cereal already full of sugar did not affect the children!

Of course, most of us know that many breakfast cereals have so much sugar that they should really be called candy. Some of these so-called food items have sugar in many forms (to trick the parent into thinking that it isn't sugar?). Sugar, whether called sucrose or fructose or any of the many other names it goes by, is still sugar to the body.

I have been around young children at birthday parties and elsewhere for over forty years. I can tell you that the effects of sugar manifest about twenty minutes after ingestion by the child. Most ECE (Early Childhood Education) people agree that the sugary birthday cakes need to be given to the children just before a recess so that the hyperactivity spike can be run off. Most of us in the ECE field dread times when the sugar is handed out right before a long bus ride.

In fact, real research (not sponsored by the sugar companies) says: "Research published in respected pediatric journals has established that sugar increases hyperactive behavior causing children to be jumpy and cranky."[134] Another book, *Taming the C.A.NDY. Monster,* was written in 1978. At that time, a "family of four consumed over 450 pounds of sugar additives in a year if their diet was typical." [135] I would venture to say that amount has skyrocketed in the intervening years.

That much sugar in the body taxes the body's ability to deal with it. The blood stream does not recognize the pancreatic secretions (insulin), the pancreas begins to not do its job, and eventually diabetes can be a result.

We get a lot more sugar than we realize because sugar hides in the most amazing places! "Most sodas, sauces, crackers, cakes, sherbets and ice creams—as well as cereals, breads, dressings and drinks—have sugar added."[136] Also, spaghetti sauce, catsup, dips, and many other items have hidden sugar.

There is no physiological requirement for refined sugar that cannot be satisfied by other, more nutritious, foods. And no authority will claim that a sugar-free diet is dangerous. ...Sugar offers no vitamins, minerals or trace elements. This refined carbohydrate is used by your body as energy or stored as fat. It does not contribute to growing strong and healthy bodies.[137]

Label reading is an important skill in trying to help your children with ADHD to become the most they can be.

> Throw out all sugar. It is an artificial food that should never have been manufactured. ...Read the labels before buying food; purchase nothing that has sugar, dextrose, or sweeteners included in the first five items on the label. ...Have no jams, jellies, canned fruit with syrup, pie, cake, cookies (or anything baked with sugar), ice cream, pop, syrup, molasses, or brown sugar in the house.[138]

Think that would be hard? Then you and your family are probably eating too much of it! You might see a dramatic change in your child's behavior and school work if you made the change: "Sometimes simply removing sugar, white flour, milk, food additives, and food colorings is sufficient to produce such a change that nothing else needs to be done."[139]

4. WHAT ABOUT ADDITIVES? DO THEY AFFECT LEARNING?

> "There is no risk with the [Feingold] diet. If the diet is tried, strict compliance must be observed—it cannot be a partial trial."
>
> Dr. Ben Feingold

Dr. Ben Feingold writes in his book, *Why Your Child is Hyperactive* that additives not only affect learning but also cause a broad range of behavioral, physiological, and neurological disturbances. Additives seem to affect many children. Additives include preservatives to keep food fresh long after it should decay if it were alive; red dye to make meat more red and, therefore, more appealing; those infamous sugar additives; and many more.

Dr. Feingold wrote *The Feingold Cookbook for Hyperactive Children* in 1979, and its premises are still being upheld today. In it, he states,

> There are now growing numbers of success stories, often dramatic, in response to dietary management. Instead of distraught parents and a disrupted home, the family life is now serene and happy; instead of conflict with peers, the children enjoy the companionship of playmates; instead of failure and frustration at school, the children's scholastic performance is not only satisfactory but frequently reported as excellent. All this is achieved without the crutch of medication, which masks the underlying condition and cures nothing.[140]

He defines foods that can have an affect on behavior as Group I or Group II. Group I is made up of all foods that contain synthetic (artificial) colors and synthetic (artificial) flavors, as well as two preservatives—the antioxidants butylated hydroxytoluen (BHT) and butylated hydroxyanisole (BHA).

Group II comprises a number of fruits and vegetables that contain natural salicylates. These include almonds, apples, apricots, berries, cloves, coffee, cucumbers and pickles, currants, grapes and raisins, to name a few.[141] Dr. Feingold eliminates all of the Group I and Group II items and this, he says, helps the children to have dramatic decreases in their ADHD symptoms.

He also suggests that nursing mothers should observe the Feingold Diet, since food additives are stored in the breast milk, are secreted when the child nurses, and can then cause disturbances in the infant.

5. WHY IS IT EVEN IMPORTANT FOR ME TO MAKE CHANGES IN MY CHILDREN'S DIET?

"Your choice of diet can influence your long-term health prospects more than any other action you might take."

Former Surgeon General C. Everett Koop

If you live with an ADHD child, you may not believe my next statement: there are other health risks besides ADHD to think of. Quoting from my dissertation, "Children's early nutrition experiences affect the rest of their life."

As stated in *First 20 Years is Life's Key to Cancer Risk,* "Lifestyle during the first 20 years of life is a more important factor than genetics when defining the risk of cancer."[142] Lifestyle diseases are on the rise because of the eating habits of adults. Those habits began in the early years and are either good or bad nutritionally.

We need not worry about how the young child will learn to eat in more healthy ways.

"A person's food preferences, like his or her personality, are formed during the first few years of life through a process of socialization. Toddlers can learn to enjoy hot and spicy food, bland health food, or fast food, depending upon what the people around them eat."[143]

Surprisingly, I found during my research that the "cause and effect" aspect of nutritionally effective eating was not clear to the mothers in the study. This is evident by the fact that many had the knowledge that animal products can cause heart disease, stroke, cancer, and many other diseases, but the mothers did not use that knowledge to cut down on those food items, let alone eliminate them.

Despite the many studies showing what a healthy diet consists of, there is less and less healthy eating in America. Some negative changes in the American diet were found on John Robbins' website:

"From 1900 to 1980 fresh fruit and vegetable consumption decreased from 40% to 5%. From 1900 to 1980 cheese consumption increased 400%. From 1900 to 1980, poultry consumption increased 350%."[144]

When one sees statistics like these, it is not surprising at all that children in America are less healthy today than they were years ago. The lack of fiber when eating a disproportionate amount of animal products certainly is a contributing factor to disease in America.

6. WHAT HEALTH HABITS DON'T DIRECTLY AFFECT LEARNING BUT ARE PART OF A HEALTHY LIFESTYLE?

"The greatness of a nation can be judged by the way its animals are treated."

Mahatma Gandhi

In order to understand a healthy diet, we should back up a bit and have a lesson on regeneration versus degeneration.

THE PHILOSOPHY OF REGENERATION IS:

- *The Body Has The Ability To Create Health And Balance When Given The Proper Nutrition.* —"The human body has considerable power to heal itself."[145] "The human body is self-repairing, self-healing, and self-maintaining, and as a matter of course, persistently martials its forces in a tireless quest to achieve and maintain health."[146]

- *This Nutrition Must Come From Whole Foods.*— "Vitamins and minerals, selectively taken from foods and put into capsules or tablets, were actually missing many of the other complex nutrients found in the original foods. Simply, it is better to eat the whole food, raw if possible and organically grown preferably, for superior good health."[147]

- *Each Individual Must Be Willing To Take Responsibility For His/*

her Own Health.— "When it comes to prevention …it's not one action that you perform. It's the way you choose to live your life! You can either live in a manner that opens the way for cancer to develop or you can live in a manner that significantly reduces your risk of it ever occurring."[148] "Health is not static. It is an ongoing condition of constant improvement."[149]

IN ADDITION, THE BODY HAS 3 BASIC NEEDS:

- *To Be Nourished*— "Naturopaths have long extolled the value of eating high-fiber foods; reducing the intake of refined sugars, fats, and food additives; exercising on a regular basis; taking nutritional supplements; and reducing stress."[150]

- *To Be Balanced*— "During a person's life, all our organs are working in concert with one another."[151]

- *To Be Cleansed*— "The inside of your body must be cleansed regularly or it will become silted up …If there is, in fact, such a thing as a 'secret' or 'key' to health, the cleansing of the inner body is surely it."[152]

Although some of the above quotations come from *You CAN Prevent Breast Cancer,* the same rules apply to other issues of health, from heart disease to other cancers. After all, health is health, and the body parts are all connected.

If any one of the above six elements is missing, the body can become out of balance and be unable to regenerate. Many people today are not nourishing the body; they are only filling it. Empty calories in the form of sugar, fat, white flour, etc. do not nourish or feed the body at the cellular level. "What most people eat today is a radical departure from what will promote good health."[153]

"Foods, every day foods, can either put us in a coffin and nail it shut or stimulate and sustain us with vibrant good health and well-being."[154]

Actually, at this point in time, most Americans' bodies are, as a result of their poor food choices, out of balance. The five main systems of the body—circulatory, immune, digestive, endocrine, and respiratory—work together in a healthy body, but they act quite differently in a body out of balance and can even attack themselves. An example is lupus.

Our collective incorrect mindset about our health affects young and old alike.

Young people seem to think that what the outside looks like at the age of 15 indicates health. But if you build a wall out of crumbly bricks and use library paste for mortar, it might look like a great wall for a short time. However, when it's 20 or 30 years old, that wall is going to start crumbling. In the same way, bones and muscles that are built out of junk food aren't going to last as long as those built out of the best food available.[155]

"And older Americans seem to think that they are immune to the laws of nature. They act as if they can violate those laws for years but not pay the price. People have been convinced that they can regularly live a life, the only possible consequence being ill health, and then run to the doctor for a pill or shot that will make everything OK, as if all past transgressions can be swept away by some potion. That's delusionary thinking that ultimately leads to one's demise.[156]

Of course, this attitude—a pill can fix anything—has been exacerbated by doctors and their "symptom-stomping" techniques.

Our medical establishment's fixation on drugs, surgery, and other high-tech interventions at the expense of low-cost preventive approaches is perhaps most evident in its failure to fully appreciate the important role of nutrition in health.[157]

"In our current medical system, not only can drugs and surgery be harmful, but so can inappropriate medications and procedures."[158]

In fact, "many drug treatments are effective only in suppressing the symptoms, whereas many natural treatments actually address the cause."[159]

Thus, a more natural approach to our lifestyle would promote health.

Now let's move on to what habits promote good health. It always amazes me that many mainstream organizations promote eating more fruits and vegetables, yet if a person chooses to eat only fruits and vegetables, that person is somehow weird or fanatic. However, in my research for both my thesis and my dissertation, it became quite clear that a vegetarian lifestyle is beneficial; and that whole foods are what the body needs.

Sharon Yntema in *Vegetarian Children* says, "Raising a child on a healthy vegetarian diet is one of the most concrete actions of love a parent can make."[160] Now let's clear some things up—catsup is not a vegetable, and neither is chocolate!

Dr. Benjamin Spock states in the forward to Dr. Attwood's book,

The evidence has been accumulating for years—from the examination of the hearts of children and young people who have died in accidents—that the process of gradual blocking of the coronary arteries begins not in adulthood but in childhood, even as young as the preschool years; and also that the main cause of this arteriosclerosis (hardening of the arteries) is the steadily increasing amount of fat in the American diet, particularly saturated animal fats such as those found in meat, chicken, milk and cheeses.[161]

Studies show that eating animal products (especially red meat) increases the chances of obesity and clogging of the arteries, and that milk is not the health factory the dairy industry would have you believe

Logically then, a vegetarian diet rich in whole grains, legumes, and fresh fruits and vegetables is the most healthy diet. Unfortunately, as I used my research tool for my dissertation, it became clear that even though many people understood the facts presented in the previous paragraph, they did not eat as if they understood. Once again, that "cause and effect" piece seemed to be missing. Logic had little or nothing to do with it.

I am a very logical person. Tell me A + B = C and show me how; I will not only believe you, but I will act on it. Unfortunately, this is not the case for most Americans. And, the media (many times funded by the Meat and Dairy Councils) helps brainwash us with advertising (every seven minutes) about the benefits of quarter-pounders with cheese and bacon. Talk about protein overkill!

The media also manipulates our thinking with reports on news shows which are conflicting and prey on people's fears. For instance, one day a study is done which states that chocolate eliminates the body's ability to assimilate calcium. Not long after, the media is fed information about the wonderful benefits of eating chocolate. I always wait for the information about who sponsored the study before making any decision about my eating habits based on that study. My thought is that if a company or industry will benefit from a study they funded, then I would certainly question the study's findings.

Obesity is yet another concern for many. Dr. Lendon Smith stated in *Improving Your Child's Behavior Chemistry* that "fat children equal fat adults."[162] If we were only concerned with looks, this would not be a problem because we have learned to be tolerant. But "there is overwhelming evidence indicating a high relationship of obesity and diabetes and cardiovascular disease"[163]

So, obesity is not just a matter of unattractiveness, it is the cause of many other diseases and life-threatening illnesses. Many people in America have already died premature deaths caused by lifestyle diseases such as obesity. Many more will die in the future unless eating habits, and other lifestyle choices, change. In fact, "Total dollar costs and deaths from excess dietary fat far exceed costs and deaths from all forms of substance abuse, including tobacco, alcohol, and illegal drugs combined"[164]

Further research has shown that "people who are overweight at 40 are likely to die at least three years sooner than those who are slim, meaning that in terms of life expectancy, being fat during middle age is just as bad as smoking."[165]

I agree with Alice Water, Chef and Owner of Chez Panisse Restaurant:

> What you eat can change your life. Food nourishes our spirits as well as our bodies. Good food—pure and wholesome food, honestly grown, and simply cooked—may be the best hope to transform our society and our consciousness. It matters profoundly.[166]

7. WHAT FOODS SHOULD I LEAVE OUT FOR MY CHILD TO BE HEALTHIER?

> "Nearly all modern diseases could be healed by avoiding meat, sugar, and refined foods and by adhering to a simple diet consisting chiefly of brown rice and vegetables."
>
> Sagen Ishizuka, M.D. (from *Diet for a Strong Heart*)

- Ideally, leaving out all animal products is healthier for the child. As the expression goes, "Just leave out eating anything that used to have a face." An additional concern with eating animal products is that most animals have a high percentage of pesticides in their flesh; when we eat that flesh, we take those pesticides into our bodies.

If you are worried about the protein issue, remember that "meat is not necessary to ensure a supply of complete proteins."[167] Pediatrician Charles R. Attwood states in his book that

> "thirteen vitamins are needed by humans. They are A, C, D, E, K, and eight B vitamins. All are obtained in adequate amounts from a variety of vegetables, fruits, whole grains, and legumes except for vitamin B12, which is produced by bacteria in animals."[168]

He goes on to quote the China Study, in which rural Chinese children who were raised as vegans (no animal products) had no B12 lack. A provocative thought is brought up by Dr. J. Gordon,

> "Animals who are supposed to eat meat have short, fast digestive systems. Instead, we have 25 feet of intestines in a system that works very slowly. We were designed to digest high-carbohydrate foods, not high-protein, high-fat meals."[169]

The logical conclusion seems to be that the meat sits around in the colon and putrefies, thus contributing to colon cancer and other health challenges.

Another concern is the connection between the hormones in beef and subsequent cancer. According to one study, "consumption of hormone treated beef may cause girls to reach puberty earlier, thus making them more susceptible to breast and other cancers."[170] Carlos Sonnenschein from Tufts University School of Medicine adds,

> Early onset of puberty with its raging hormones translates into higher risk of breast cancer and it is very likely that hormone residues in North American beef are a contributing factor in the early onset of puberty among girls observed in recent decades.[171]

• Dairy is especially important to leave out because:

> Excess amounts of proteins—especially of animal proteins—cause changes in kidney activity, resulting in large losses of calcium from the body. Experimental studies show that protein levels commonly consumed by Americans—90 grams and more, 15% of the calories—will cause more calcium to be lost from the body than can be absorbed from the gut, even when the person is consuming very high levels of calcium.[172]

• Leave out all hydrogenated oils, also called trans-fats, which you will find in many products. Staying away from trans-fats will help in the battle against the buildup of plaque on the artery walls.

• Leave out sugar. *Ahrgh-h-h-h*…I can hear you! But,

> give a toddler sugar for breakfast, you'll have a morning of "terrible twos" behavior ahead of you. A snack of sweet, milky cocoa with marshmallows and cookies will mean a fidgety child for the rest of the afternoon. And the child who eats sugar before bedtime will probably be cranky, whining, and awake two hours later.[173]

There are perfectly acceptable substitutes for sugar that don't harm the pancreas, such as stevia. Stevia is 300 times sweeter than sugar, so it isn't as expensive as it seems at first glance. "Stevia is a healthy, delicious alternative to sugars and artificial sweeteners. Delicious, that is, if you use a recipe designed for stevia."[174] Stevia kills yeast, so it's a good food for those with Candida. Killing the yeast, though, is not so great if you want the bread to rise!

- Leave out white flour, grind your own! Fresh, ground, whole wheat flour has many nutrients, micronutrients, and phytochemicals not found in store-bought bread. It takes only an extra minute or two to grind your own wheat. And there are many recipes that taste so much better when they are made with freshly ground whole wheat. With the new bread makers, making your own bread only takes about five minutes; the bread maker does all the hard parts. Yea!

- Leave out processed foods as much as possible. They usually have the fiber and nutrients processed right out of them and lots of chemical preservatives put in.

  The processed food industry concentrates on addicting them to dead, chemicalized foods so they will eat them from morning until night. In spite of the efforts of many aware parents to eliminate dead foods from their children's diets, advertising continuously pushes these poisons on the kids.[175]

- Leave out cooking at high temperatures.

  Many fast food restaurants cook high-fat meat with high fat cooking methods, often over a grill. The result is that fat falls on the hot flame and creates increased free radicals in the food. These unstable oxygen molecules are charcoal-like compounds which raise blood pressure, increase heart disease, and promote the incidence of cancer.[176]

- Leave out hot dogs! "I feel there's nothing wrong with telling a child that hot dogs are filled with pig lips and cow ears."[177]

- Leave out TV and hand-held game playing. The medical journal *Pediatrics* published a provocative study looking at television-viewing habits of about 2,600 children ages one to three. The researchers found that the more television children were exposed to at a young age, the more likely their parents were to report attention problems at age 7."[178]

I would venture to say that this is because when children use hand-held games and watch a lot of TV, they don't get the cross-lateral activity necessary to build dendrites in the brain. And, they need *lots* of cross-lateral activity (opposite arm and opposite leg) in order to build those dendrites! Cross-lateral activities also help adults' and children's ADHD symptoms. Examples of cross-lateral activity are walking and running.

If you're still worried about making these changes, consider the five-year Children's Achievement Program for Educational Readiness. In this long-term study, the participants received diet education and nutritional support, in which highly refined foods and sugars were sharply reduced and replaced by fresh fruits and vegetables and whole-wheat flour. Chocolate milk, sugar-coated breakfast cereals, and sugared doughnuts were eliminated in preference for healthier eating choices. Those who had reached the fifth or sixth grade were found to have an accelerated performance in school and were at or above their regular designated grade levels at the completion of the program. This study shows that even modest changes toward a more healthful diet are beneficial.

8. WHERE DO I START WHEN BUYING HEALTHIER FOODS?

"Before you can change your eating habits…you will have to change your buying habits."

Sharon Yntema

First, and foremost, stop buying anything that is processed. If you are extremely frugal and just can't see yourself going home and throwing away "good" (I say that advisedly) food, then use up what you have and just don't buy anymore. Offer only healthy foods and do not give in to the whining for the junk foods the children are used to eating. As you go through the transition, keep reminding yourself that you "loved them enough" as Erma Bombeck wrote.

Secondly, read all the labels. You will be amazed at how many items have sugar, hydrogenated oils, preservatives, or other unhealthy ingredients. If they have these items, don't buy them.

Thirdly, begin reading every book available on how to change to a more healthy diet. Many of them have sections which help with the transition stage. For instance, in the book *Vegetarian Children, a Supportive Guide for Parents,*[179] Sharon Yntema has a transitional buying guide which is very helpful. It shows what to cut out—baked goods with refined flours and sugar—and what to add—rice cakes, whole-grain breads.

Save money by making homemade meals (which are usually lower in all the bad ingredients such as hydrogenated oils, sugar, processing, and preservatives). I live a very busy life, but most of my meals are homemade.

I began using my crock-pot, along with a "cooking for an army" thought-process; I now have a different homemade meal every day. Here's how I do it: whenever I have time, I make a huge batch of something. It could be pinto beans, spaghetti sauce, split pea soup, chili, or thirteen bean soup. I freeze it in containers that hold enough for a meal. Each morning I decide what I want for dinner; I take it out of the freezer, pop it out of the container, and then put it into the crockpot on low for dinner. At whatever time I come home, the house smells wonderful and I can eat right then if I'm hungry. This eliminates that "grab junk because I'm starving" syndrome.

One of my favorite recipes is Four Season Savory Stew found in *CalciYum*.[180] This stew has lots of calcium, lots of taste, and a beautiful golden color.

Sometimes I combine three or four containers from the freezer to make a brand new type of soup. Just recently, I added my home-fries to the split pea soup I was making, and it was delicious. In fact, I was working on the final phase of this manuscript with Dr. Parslow, and she said it was the best soup she'd ever tasted! Check *www.ececonsultants.com* for my cookbook containing this recipe.

9. SHOULD I LOOK INTO ORGANIC FOODS AND, IF SO, WHY?

"Why sneaky? Well, sneaky cookery is the art of incorporating into every dish the food values—the vitamins and minerals and enzymes—that would have been there in the first place if the food had not been processed, devitalized, and loaded with additives and thus stripped of much of its nutritive value."

Jane Kinderlehrer
(author of *Confessions of a Sneaky Organic Cook*)

In *Poisoning Our Children*, Nancy Sokol Green gives us some information about the pesticides located in all non-organic foods. She began learning about the chemicals all around us when she became ill and was, finally, diagnosed as chemically sensitive or environmentally ill.

She found that thirty different pesticides have been found in carrots alone. One was DDT. Even though it's been banned since 1972, it is still in the soil and therefore gets into the food chain. Dieldrin (another banned pesticide) has also been detected in produce. She writes, "It is known to cause birth defects and reproductive toxicity in animal studies. Even low levels have caused learning disabilities in monkeys."[181]

She continues, "Carrots are not singled out. Every non-organic fruit and vegetable may contain multiple numbers of pesticide residues."[182]

This is disturbing, and one might decide to do a better job of washing those veggies. However, she writes,

> In most cases, washing produce will not eliminate pesticide residues for several reasons. First, most pesticides are specifically formulated to be water resistant since farmers and growers do not want their pesticide application to be washed away with the first rain. Second, many pesticides are systemic, making any outside scrubbing futile.[183]

In addition, produce that has been waxed also poses a concern since waxing seals in pesticide residues, to say nothing of the fungicide added to the wax itself.

> While most consumers may know that cucumbers are waxed, they may not know that a number of other fruits and vegetables are also routinely waxed. These include apples, avocados, bell peppers, cantaloupes, eggplants, grapefruits, lemons, limes, melons, oranges, parsnips, passion fruits, peaches, pineapples, pumpkins, rutabagas, squash, sweet potatoes and turnips.[184]

Imported foods contain much higher percentages of pesticides than is allowed for foods grown in the U.S., so many companies import their food. Does this make sense to you?

> Up to 70% of the food grown abroad with the aid of unregistered, banned or severely restricted pesticides is exported back into this country.....The fact that so much of the food grown abroad gets exported back to this country calls into question the argument that hazardous pesticides are desperately needed by Third World countries so that they can grow food to alleviate hunger.
>
> The fact is that there is enough food in the world for everyone. But tragically, much of the world's food and land resources are tied up in producing beef and other livestock—food for the well-off—while

millions of children and adults suffer from malnutrition and starvation.[185]

Organic fruits and vegetables take one detrimental item away from the food table and should be seriously considered by the person wanting to be healthier. For an excellent fruit and vegetable mix that provides, in one tablespoon, the benefits of five plates of dark leafy greens, see www.ececonsultants.com.

10. WHICH IS BETTER? SIMPLE, RAW, ORGANIC FOODS OR PROCESSED, COOKED FOODS

"The raw food diet goes well beyond the physical body. It changes us at an energetic and cellular level."

Cheryl Stoycoff (author: *Raw Kids*)

One of the simplest, but hardest, choices to make is to eat all raw foods. For many, the cooked food is so addictive that they never quite make it to a "raw food" table. The reasons can be many, but the need to smell the food as it is cooked is the most difficult for me.

However, the benefits of eating raw foods are numerous. First, the enzymes in the food are not killed by cooking, so more nutrition is available to the body. Further, there are no hydrogenated oils in raw fruits or vegetables, thus eliminating a major health risk. They also have no cholesterol. If you use organic foods, there are no pesticides. Natural, fresh, organic fruits and vegetables have no preservatives in them either.

The difficulty in moving towards a raw diet brings up my philosophy about making changes: every step in the right direction counts. Even baby steps! I did not become vegan overnight; I cut out red meat, then poultry, then fish, and finally dairy. I am now working on adding more and more raw foods into my diet. I am so much healthier today because of those baby steps.

Guilt is not part of my lifestyle. I do as much as I can as fast as I can.

11. HOW CAN I MAKE MY LIFE AND ENVIRONMENT HEALTHIER?

"A report by the United States Department of Agriculture estimates that 89 percent of U.S. beef ground into patties contains traces of the deadly E. coli strain."

Reuters News Service

You probably don't have to go to the extremes that Nancy Sokol Green has because of her sensitivity. She had to sell her home, which was toxic. She had to buy a different home and be sure that it had never had chemicals put onto the lawn or into the house. Then she had the carpet and linoleum ripped up and then made sure the glue for the new wood floors would not be toxic. Even if you don't go that far, it is important to become more aware of the chemicals around you.

For instance, have you thought about the ingredients in your acrylic fingernails? Or the glue that holds on your plastic ones? Have you thought about the bi-monthly sprayings on your lawn or chemicals in your home? Have you considered the fact that many schools spray the classrooms with the children right in them? Some of those chemical sprays contain the same ingredient as Agent Orange!

The everyday environment that your children live in can be toxic and contribute to their mental and physical challenges. As shown by Nancy Sokol Green, you and your children are exposed to thousands of pesticides and other toxins every single day. In fact, each day we are exposed to more toxins than our ancestors were exposed to in an entire lifetime! New carpets outgas (outgassing is the slow release of a gas that was trapped, frozen, or absorbed in the material), glues used on floorings are toxic to many, and there are many other issues.

Becoming aware and being an activist is so very important. In America, we seem to think that "big brother" is watching over us and keeping us safe. This is *not* the case. For instance, chemical spray companies are businesses trying to make money; whatever way they can convince you that you need their service is, to them, acceptable.

12. HOW CAN I HELP MY CHILDREN SEE A CAUSE AND EFFECT RELATIONSHIP BETWEEN WHAT THEY EAT AND THEIR FUTURE HEALTH?

"When you see the Golden Arches, you're probably on the road to the pearly gates."

Dr. William Castelli, M.D., Director,
Framingham Health Study

I've mentioned the lack of the "cause and effect" mentality; it is one of the most disturbing aspects of my dissertation research.

The researcher also found that the "cause and effect" aspect of nutritionally effective eating, was not clear to the mothers in the study. This is clearly shown by the fact that many had the knowledge that animal products can cause heart disease, stroke, cancer and many other diseases but the mothers did not use that knowledge to cut down on those food items. Despite the many studies showing what a healthy diet consists of, there is less and less healthy eating in America.[186]

SOME IDEAS TO HELP

Since you are reading this, I can assume that you are interested in your children's health, so here are some ideas to help.

- Don't live mindlessly. Be a thinker, be a questioner. Don't just do or eat what everyone else in America is doing or eating.

- The most important activity you can do with and for your children's eventual lifestyle habits is to be a good role model. You are the biggest influence in your children's lives. If you eat junk foods, it's going to be hard to convince your children to eat in healthy ways.

- Have only healthy foods in your house. Do not think you are doing your child a favor to give in to their nagging for junk foods. Remember the acronym for candy is Continuously Advertised Nutritionally Deficient Yummies. You are actually showing how much you love your child by **not** giving in!

- If your children refuse to eat a healthy dinner and then carry on at bedtime for ice cream, you are not showing them true love by giving in. If you've lived your life differently until now, it may take some time to convince your children that you are serious about helping them be healthy. But if you are absolutely convinced that you are doing the right thing, then stand your ground! You can tell them: "Life is full of changes, and we are changing to a healthier lifestyle. So, welcome to a new chapter in our family book!"

- Never use sweets to reward; this is so counterproductive! Behaving should not be rewarded with sweets ("You were so good, I'll give you this candy".) Neither should misbehaving ("If you quiet down, I'll give you a candy".)

- This one is probably my biggest issue: Holiday get-togethers with friends or family are special because of the people we see, not the amount of sweets we eat. Create traditions having to do with the people instead of the junk food and sweets.

- The last idea is probably the very best. Verbalize what you learn as you do your own research on healthy eating habits. Parents are the very first teachers of children, and children will learn if you help teach them.

You are in the perfect position to affect your child's entire life. Yea! And, the above Twelve Step Questions will help you. If you have questions or just need more information, I would love to mentor you on this adventure, just contact me!

Note: The previous article by Dr. Carroll forms the basis for her soon to be published book on children's health. You can reach her at the address below. Available on the website are many products to help you in your quest for better health. (Ellouise@ececonsultants.com) or *www.ececonsultants.com.*

30 Pregnancy Tips

"Now that you are pregnant, let's put you on prenatal vitamins." So said my obstetrician many years back when I was expecting my first child. I obliged him by taking the one-a-day pill. "Just eat a balanced diet," he said. But he never asked me what I ate, so how would he know if it was balanced? My husband and I always had fairly healthy meals. But I also ate lots of fast foods, junk foods, soft drinks, candy, and pastries. My diet also included plenty of airline food since I was a flight attendant at the time. Shortly thereafter, my journey to a healthier life began when I wandered into a health food store and the owner gave me some carrot juice. I learned much from her and by my second pregnancy, I knew a lot more about healthy eating!

THE EXTRAORDINARY WORK OF WESTON PRICE, D.D.S.

The extraordinary work of the late Weston Price, D.D.S. (1870–1948), as recorded in *Nutrition and Physical Degeneration*, demonstrates that what a mother eats prior to and during pregnancy directly affects the health of her unborn child. Dr. Price left his dental practice at the age of sixty to travel the world with his wife and study what he called "primitive civilizations."

His research clearly established that cultures eating their native diets of natural, whole, unadulterated foods produced children in good health with strong physiques and broad jaws, with plenty of room for their perfectly formed, resilient teeth.

His book and historic video are available through the Price-

Pottenger Foundation at www.price-pottenger.org. Every person who is interested in the health of their family or the critical lack of health in our nation should get this video and share it with others.

Clearly, the time to start good nutrition for your child is before you become pregnant. Your diet should be rich in nutrient-dense whole foods, protein, and folic acid-rich foods like dark, leafy-green vegetables. Your doctor will most likely recommend a high quality vitamin/mineral supplement, but don't count on it completely. Follow a whole, natural diet as outlined in this book.

FISH, MERCURY, & PREGNANCY

While fish contains high-quality protein and omega-3 fatty acids, nearly all fish and shellfish contain traces of mercury.

> Mercury is a contaminant found in fish that can affect brain development and the nervous system. The FDA has released guidelines for women who are pregnant and women who are trying to become pregnant. These guidelines state that no more than 12 oz. of low mercury fish should be consumed weekly. "Highest" mercury fish should be avoided and "high" mercury fish should be kept to only three 6-oz. servings per month.[187]

A WORD ON BREASTFEEDING

While reports most often emphasize the positive benefits of breast-feeding for the infant, recent studies reveal important benefits for the nursing mother. Here is a recent report on breast cancer:

> A 2002 study published in the British Medical Journal, *The Lancet*, collaboratively analyzed individual data from 47 studies in 30 countries, including 50,302 women with breast cancer and 96,973 without

the disease. The study found that a woman's risk for breast cancer decreased by 4.3 percent for every 12 months she breastfed during her lifetime. The risk also decreased 7 percent for every child born. According to the data, breast cancer in some African and Asian countries is relatively uncommon compared to cases in the United States and many countries in Europe. The difference is that women in less developed countries have many more children and breastfeed much longer than their counterparts in developed countries.[188]

THE SAFE AND SENSIBLE USE OF HERBS

3 **1** The Safe and Sensible Use of Herbs

My interest in natural health actually began in my early thirties when *Herbally Yours* by Penny Royal ended up in my hands. At the time, I was a flight attendant and had just come out of the hospital where I had been in traction for a back injury resulting from a cross-country flight.

The book talked about valerian root, an herb that was good for relieving pain. It said that the drug Valium was fashioned after it. I thought I might be able to use it instead of the painkillers given to me by the doctor. I bought some valerian root at the health food store and it worked.

This sparked my interest; I continued reading and learned that nature has a whole array of healing herbs. I read that marshmallow wasn't just a soft, sweet treat, but was an herb good for hay fever. That nineteenth century physicians whipped up a foamy meringue from the marshmallow root juices, added egg white and honey, and gave the hardened candy to soothe children's sore throats.

That book changed the whole trajectory of my life. Shortly after reading it, with confidence running high, I ran into a woman whose husband had a problem.

A STORE OWNER'S STORY

"THAT COMFREY HEALED HIS FOOT ULCER WHEN MEDICATION WOULDN'T"

I was ordering little league trophies for my oldest son's team. The owner of the store told me that her husband had a diabetic ulcer on his foot that his doctors had not been able to heal. Knowing just a little about herbs, I told her I had read that the herb comfrey had a substance in it called *allantoin* that was said to be a wound healer. Then on my way I went.

When I went back to pick up the trophies, she told me that she had immediately bought comfrey at her local health food store. She had made a poultice (a bandage large enough to cover the affected area with the moistened herb in it) for his sore and applied it several times a day.

"That comfrey healed his foot ulcer when medication wouldn't. When he went in for follow-up treatment, I told the doctor we were using it, and he said it was okay, and that it couldn't hurt anything."

———

Since that experience, I've always kept herbs of all sorts on hand. They have many uses for common ailments and can often be combined with medical orders from a qualified healthcare practitioner to speed healing.

Do not stop using your prescribed medication. Herbs should always be used under the direction of a qualified health practitioner.

THE HISTORY OF HERBAL USE

For centuries, herbs have been recognized as natural remedies for treating various diseases. With the rise in popularity of modern medicine, they fell by the wayside, but in recent years, there has been a renewed interest in their use.

> In the United States, herbal remedies were used widely until the early 1900s when what was to become the modern pharmaceutical industry began. Medicine became almost exclusively committed to a medical system some practitioners call *allopathy*, which seeks to treat illness by producing a condition in the body that does not allow the disease to live or thrive. Over the years, most Americans have become conditioned to rely on synthetic, commercial drugs for relief.[189]

However, the World Health Organization has estimated that 80% of the world's population may rely on "traditional" medicines for their primary health care needs. Since herbal medicine is a large portion of traditional therapies, is can be assumed that the majority of the people in the world use plants as medicines. [190]

HOW HERBS ARE FORMULATED & TAKEN

Herbal preparations are available in all sorts of venues—bulk herbs, teas, capsules, lotions, tinctures, blends, and extracts.

Herbs fall into two basic categories: *tonic* and *stimulating*. The tonics help the cells and tissues maintain tone and are used for months at a time to gently strengthen and improve overall health or the health of certain organs.

Stimulating herbs are used to treat particular ailments and are generally used for shorter periods of time in smaller doses.

Salves, ointments, and *creams* contain specifically selected herbs mixed with an oily base. They are used externally on the skin. Syrups are used internally and are often sweetened to hide the taste of the herb. Cough syrups are an example.

Teas, also called *infusions,* are made from various parts of the plant like bark, roots, leaves, seeds, or berries.

Essential oils, also known as *volatile* oils, are highly concentrated extracts from various parts of plants. They contain many natural ingredients from the plant such as vitamins, antibiotics, and natural, hormone-like substances. They are used topically, in baths, as inhalants, or as poultices. Oils are available for most conditions—from arthritis and respiratory discomfort to toothache and headaches.

KATRINA'S STORY

"THIS NAGGING PAIN IS MORE THAN I CAN DEAL WITH"

"On September 10, 2003, a wonderful birth took place, that of my first born son. However, in the midst of this most joyous occasion, I was overwhelmed by immense postpartum pain. I had torn horribly during the delivery process and had to be stitched back together. Nothing relieved my pain!

I had natural childbirth and could handle that, but I was now in constant pain, which I could not seem to overcome. I tried a few over-the-counter medications and readily available pain relievers, but they did nothing to alleviate my suffering. They just made me tired. So for the first week, I stayed on the couch—in pain.

When I tried to get up and walk to my son, I could barely waddle even a short distance before needing to sit and rest. I'd given birth naturally, and now this constant nagging pain was more than I could deal with! I was praying that somehow I could find relief.

Relief arrived! My father (Ron Lowrie, contributing author) had a few tricks in his biblical apothecary satchel when he showed up about a week and a half into my dilemma. He suggested I use an all natural essential oil combination that was a mixture of clove, helichrysum (from Italian everlasting plant), birch, and peppermint.

I will admit it did burn a little, but it was nothing compared to the unbearable pain I had been experiencing. Within minutes, I was finally able to walk comfortably after just one application. He also suggested a spray made from the herb lavender to help refresh and calm the wounded and swollen area.

Within about a week, I was finally walking around the house and caring for my little bundle of joy. I say thanks to God for His universal laws of health and vitality available through His miraculous plant kingdom."

——

Most likely, Katrina got relief because the herbs had strong anti-inflammatory properties. If the subject of herbs interests you (as it did me well over two decades ago), begin reading! Most likely, you'll find the answers you are looking for at your library, in natural food book sections, or on the internet.

Now that you understand a little about herbs, let's take a look at commonly used choices.

③②　Healing Benefits of Eighteen Commonly Used Herbs

ALFALFA

Alfalfa has been referred to as "the father of all foods." The roots grow deep into the earth, making the leaves rich in calcium, magnesium, potassium, and vitamins A, D, E, and K.

Traditionally used as an immune-system enhancer, a few other benefits include easing arthritic pain, lowering cholesterol, and clearing and detoxifying the liver. Some scientific studies say that the chemicals in alfalfa lower cholesterol and help decrease its absorption.

Alfalfa is available in tablets, liquid drops, and as tea. It is also an excellent addition to the diet in the form of sprouts. Try the sprouts on sandwiches, salads, or sprinkled on main dishes. Because alfalfa sprouts can be moldy, always wash them before eating.

ALOE VERA

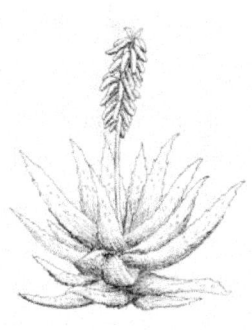

Aloe Vera leaves contain a pulp on the inside that can be used topically to heal burns. Many burn ointments have aloe vera as a main ingredient. Aloe can be taken by mouth in the form of juice, gels, and capsules and is known to lower cholesterol, increase poor circulation, and act as a laxative. It is also good for digestive disorders and is used in many anti-aging facial formulas. Various kinds of aloe are available at *www. gethealthyamerica.biz.*

AVA LEE'S ALOE STORY

"ALOE VERA GOT RID OF TEETH PLAQUE"

Years ago, my mother told me that a coworker suffered with thick, heavy plaque on her teeth. A friend gave her some toothpaste with aloe vera in it, and she began to use it daily. On her next visit to her dentist, he exclaimed, "What have you done to your teeth? You have no plaque on them!"

Note: You may also find it effective to gargle with aloe juice or rub the inside of fresh leaves on the gums and teeth after brushing.

BLACK COHOSH

This herb is known to balance hormones in men and women and is used in the treatment of symptoms of menopause, PMS, and related hormonal problems. It should not be used during pregnancy. It is available in tincture and capsules.

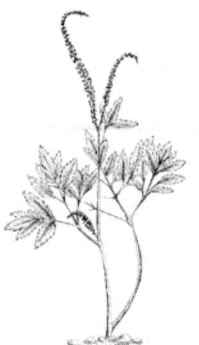

Many of the earliest patent medicines contained high concentrations of black cohosh. It was the main ingredient in "Lydia Pinkham's Vegetable Compound", an over-the-counter remedy promoted in the early 19th century as relieving stress and nervous tension in women. It has become the best selling herb in the world for treatment of menstrual problems. Ten million units of a single brand, Remifemin, are sold monthly in Australia, Germany, and the United States.[191]

CAYENNE (CAPSICUM)

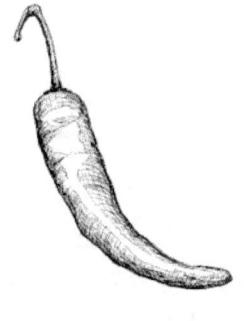

Cayenne is known to aid digestion and improve circulation. It is beneficial for the heart and stomach. In one study conducted on medical students in Bangkok, researchers fortified rice noodles with freshly ground capsicum peppers. They gave some of the medical students the peppery noodles. The others had only plain noodles. Almost immediately, the pepper-laced noodle eaters showed clot-dissolving activity in their blood. The high consumption of cayenne contributed to the lack of blood clots among the students.[192]

Tip: replace the black pepper shaker on your table with cayenne pepper. Black pepper is not from the capsicum family and does not provide the same benefits.

COMFREY

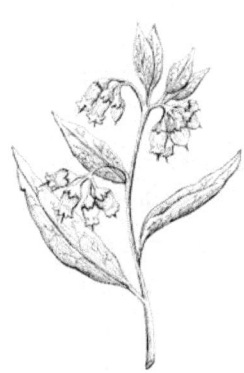

Comfrey contains an ingredient called *allantoin*, a compound that helps stimulate the growth of new cells. Comfrey was called "knitbone" by American Indians for its ability to heal bones and speed healing of wounds. The herb is good for warts, skin tags, and cuts. It should be taken internally only under medical direction.

Comfrey is excellent as a poultice. To make a poultice, cut a piece of cloth twice as large as the area you wish to cover, and use a freshly picked comfrey leaf with its root. Wash the leaf and root, crush or chop them finely, and cover with very hot water for a few minutes to activate the ingredients. Drain and place the ingredients on one side of a cloth, fold over the other half, and apply to affected part of the body. Leave the poultice in place for up to thirty minutes.

MARC'S AMAZING COMFREY STORY

"MOM! LOOK! IT'S FORMING A SCAB!"

My oldest son, Marc, had an extensive paper route when he was in the seventh grade. Since he needed to make several trips home to pick up more papers, my husband decided to weld a newspaper carrier to the back of his bike.

Very shortly thereafter, Marc saw the shiny paper carrier securely attached and ready to be filled with papers. So he ran up and plopped himself down on the seat.

The metal was still scalding hot; he singed his right, inside thigh with a burn about the size of a silver dollar. I immediately put some burn ointment on it to relieve the pain and to disinfect the wound.

I went to the kitchen cupboard where I had some comfrey herbal teabags. Knowing that the American Indians used the herb comfrey for all kinds of ailments, including burns, I decided to try it on Marc's burn.

I soaked a teabag in hot water a couple of minutes to activate the herbs, then had Marc place it on the burn. He was watching cartoons, so he obliged me by leaving it in place for about thirty minutes. Then he discarded the teabag and went back out to play. About an hour later, he burst into the front door.

"Mom! Look!" The circular burn had begun forming a scab, almost as if he'd taken a marking pen and drawn a circle completely around the burn. We were both amazed and anxious to continue the comfrey treatment. So for two days, we kept the sore clean and applied a comfrey teabag twice daily. We watched as that scab grew smaller and smaller until it popped off! And there was no visible scar. This was my first experience with herbal healing, and I will never forget it! Since that time, I've always made sure I had comfrey growing in my yard.

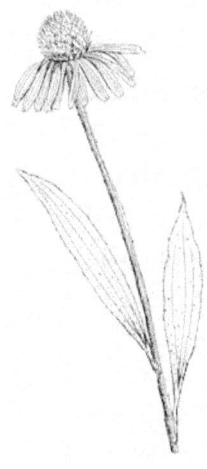

ECHINACEA

The leaves and roots of echinacea are used to fight inflammation and bacterial/viral infections. It is good for the immune system and is a popular wintertime flu-fighter in supplemental form or as a tea. It is good as a gargle for dental abscesses and effective in compresses to bathe wounds.

Echinacea is one of the most popular and well known herbs. And there are numerous scientific studies on the medicinal power, which is why so many people choose it.

Numerous studies from around the world conclude that echinacea helps cold sufferers to recover faster and experience less severity of symptoms. The herb works especially well on people with weak immune systems.

MARTHA'S ECHINACEA STORY AS TOLD BY RON LOWRIE

"I TOOK A HARD FALL ON THE ICY PAVEMENT"

I was at a winter retreat in the snowy Pacific Northwest Cascades. The hosts were Adventist friends, and the guests were from all around the United States.

Martha, an elderly attendee, took a hard fall on the icy pavement and landed on both knees. Untimely as it was, we were set for hands-on practice that day. The herbalist presenter was extremely knowledgeable in the use of natural remedies.

We observed as he cleaned the wounds with water, and then applied a thin sprinkling of echinacea powder to her bruised and bleeding knees. Next, he applied a thin coat of raw honey that would serve as a protective, anti-bacterial coating and also would reduce inflammation. Then he wrapped her knees.

Although her knees were tender, the pain in them began to subside immediately. She was able to walk up and down stairs the next day, and she enjoyed the remainder of the conference.

The Bible speaks of milk and honey. In ancient times, it was used not only as a food but also as a healing compound. Science has identified a substance called *inhibine,* which resists infection and speeds the healing process. The bees probably know how all this works, so they can keep intruders from invading their hives. Echinacea is known for its antiseptic and other healing properties, so we had a good combination. (Inhibine is a bacteria-killing agent found only in raw honey. It is destroyed during pasteurization.)[193]

FENUGREEK

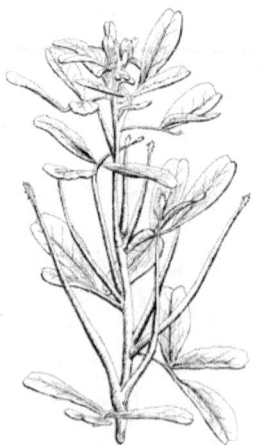

Fenugreek (Greek = plant) acts as a laxative, lubricating the intestines. It has also been used for centuries in the Middle East and India to treat several diseases, including diabetes.

Scientists at India's National Institute of Nutrition recently tested ground up fenugreek seeds on insulin-dependent diabetics. They added it to the lunch and dinner meals of several diabetics. What they found was that:

"...fenugreek dramatically reduced fasting blood sugar levels in the diabetics. It also reduced total cholesterol and triglycerides. The active ingredient in the seeds is a gel-like soluble fiber called *galactomannan.*"[194]

Since the results indicate the usefulness of fenugreek seeds in the management of diabetes, if you or someone you know is diabetic, why not add it to your diet? Thai, Indian, Middle Eastern, and Pakistani cookbooks will show you how to incorporate fenugreek. It is also available as a supplement.

FEVERFEW

As thousands of sufferers will tell you, this little herb from the daisy family works to shut off the excruciating pain of migraine headaches. Used historically for the treatment of headaches, feverfew remains commonly used today. It is available in many natural formulas. It has also been used for arthritis, menstrual discomfort, and other aches and pains.

Dr. E. Johnson of London had read that feverfew would help migraines, so he questioned almost 300 migraine headache sufferers who regularly used feverfew.

> Seventy-two percent of sufferers who chewed feverfew leaves claimed reduced occurrence and pain from their migraines. Later, he encapsulated feverfew and gave it to only some of the patients. Those receiving it were relatively migraine-free, but the patients who didn't get feverfew were in severe pain. Feverfew's secret component is *parthenolide* thought to affect blood vessel constriction.[195]

GREEN TEA

Green tea—a powerful antioxidant—is said to protect against cancer and reduce blood clotting, and it is thought to be

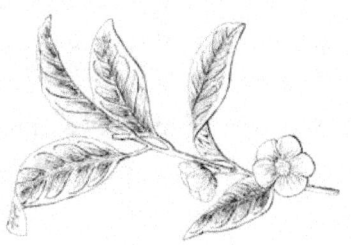

helpful in preventing an enlarged prostate. Researchers have found that a *polyphenol* in green tea (*epigallocatechin gallate-EGCG*) is 20 times more powerful than vitamin E and 200 times more powerful than vitamin C. [196] It is available in supplemental form from *www. gethealthyamerica.biz.*

GINGER

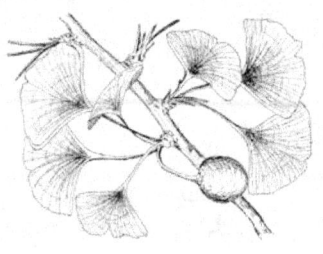

Ginger is often used to reduce spasms, cramps, nausea, and vomiting. Eighty Denmark naval cadets unaccustomed to sailing in heavy seas were given either one gram of ginger or a placebo. Ginger reduced the tendency to vomiting and cold sweats. Fewer symptoms of nausea and vertigo were reported after ginger ingestion.

GINKGO BILOBA

A favorite for improving brain function by increasing circulation and tissue oxygenation, ginkgo biloba also has antioxidant properties. It is good for age-related decrease in eye function and mental awareness, and its flavonoids act to dilate the smallest capillaries, allowing good blood flow to the body. Its medicinal use can be traced back thousands of years.

Researchers have recognized for decades that ginkgo therapy reduces the severity of symptoms of dementia and Alzheimer's due to its ability to improve glucose metabolism and increase brain oxygen. Ginkgo is available in capsules, tablets, and teas. The tea form does not provide the concentration available in capsules.

HYSSOP

Referred to numerous times in the Bible, hyssop was used historically for cleansing and purifying the body. Hippocrates, the father of medicine used it, recommending it as an anti-inflammation wash.

Other uses of hyssop include relief of lung congestion and regulation of blood pressure. It has a tonic effect on the blood, helping to open up the oxygen-receptor sites on red blood cells.

LICORICE

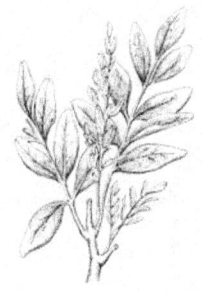

A number of studies have confirmed licorice's anti-ulcer effect, which typically equals that of prescription drugs such as Tagamet. The herb's protective effect on the liver has been confirmed by a sixteen-year study of patients with chronic hepatitis C. In this study, patients receiving a glycyrrhizin extract had a significantly lower rate of liver cancer. The soothing action of licorice has been known since antiquity.[197]

In other studies, it has been found that licorice root has formidable anti-ulcer properties. European scientists found that licorice compounds reduced acidity, stimulated mucous secretion, and helped stomach-wall cells repair themselves. *Deglycyrrhizinated licorice* (DGL) can avoid elevated blood pressure because the compound that causes this problem has been removed.

MILK THISTLE

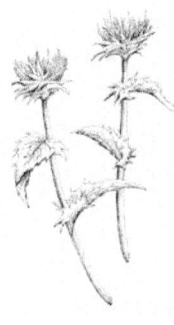

Milk thistle is an herb proven to protect the liver from toxins and pollutants by preventing free-radical damage. It has also been shown to have anti-cancer effects against prostate/breast cancer. Milk thistle is an herb commonly found in formulas for liver cleansing and is used routinely in the natural medicine field.

PARSLEY

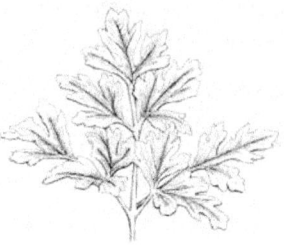

Parsley contains an ingredient known to prevent the multiplication of cancer cells. It is also beneficial to relieve gas, freshen breath, lower high blood pressure, and relieve water retention. It is very high in vitamin C. I always said to my children when we ate out, "Eat your parsley. It's the healthiest thing on your plate!" And as flight attendants, we learned to take the parsley off the dinner plates to make tea. It definitely kept the swelling out of our ankles, which is common "at altitude."

ST. JOHN'S WORT

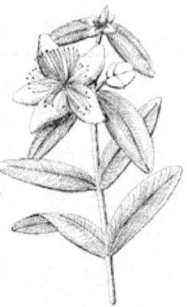

This herb has been tested extensively in Europe and is used by millions of Germans and Europeans. A common wildflower with bright yellow flowers, it contains *hypericin*, the medicinally active component. St. John's Wort is known to relieve depression.

> In a recent survey conducted in Germany on 3,250 depressed patients, nearly 80% showed improvement after a four-week trial of St. John's wort. The age of the patients ranged from 20–90 years with an average age of 51.[198]

St. John's wort is also effective as an anti-bacterial, anti-inflammatory, and for pain relief.

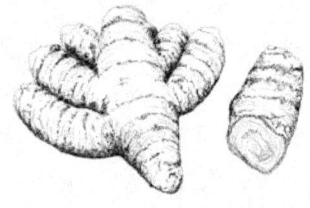

TURMERIC

The main ingredient in curry powder, turmeric fights free radicals, protects the liver against toxins, aids circulation, improves blood vessel health, stimulates bile secretion, and has antibiotic and anti-cancer properties. It is good for arthritis.

Researchers from the University of Arizona College of Medicine report that turmeric may hold promise both for the prevention of rheumatoid arthritis and osteoporosis. *Curcumin,* an ingredient in turmeric, is thought to be responsible because of its ability to turn off inflammation in joints and to slow down bone loss.[199]

WILD YAM

This herb is known to contain compounds similar to the hormone estrogen. Many yam-based products are available in natural food stores. The herb is often used by women who are premenstrual or those going through menopause. Other reported uses include relief of muscle spasms, improvement in gallbladder disorders, and reduction of inflammation. It should not be used by pregnant women.

THE VITAMINS

3 3 Vitamins A, C, D, and E

As the story goes, a well balanced diet will provide your body with all it needs to stay healthy and free of disease. You'll just need to choose daily from each of the food groups: fats, milk, vegetables, protein, fruit, and breads. That way, you will be getting all the vitamins and minerals you need. But what if you choose the correct amount of food from each food group, but your choices look like this:

- Milk Group: one highly sweetened fruit yogurt and one chocolate milk

- Vegetable Group: two servings of French fries (the number one eaten vegetable in America), an iceberg lettuce salad (very low in nutrition), and one serving of canned corn or peas

- Meat Group: one deep-fried chicken breast, batter-fried fish, or roast beef microwavable "TV dinner"

- Fruit Group: an apple

- Fat Group: margarine on a potato or salad dressing made with hydrogenated oil

- Carbohydrate Group: white bread, white rice, or white dinner roll

At this juncture in the book, you are probably realizing that the Standard American Diet is anything but balanced and that our national health statistics serve as a warning, loud and clear, that our American diet is drastically nutrient deficient.

Call it a hazard of modern, industrialized living. It has become almost impossible to get all our vitamins and minerals from our food, even when we are making the healthiest choices possible. So say scientists and numerous clinical studies—not just radical and fringy health nuts! Prestigious mainstream universities and colleges are confirming and reconfirming that adding supplements to the diet is a powerful way to fight off aging and disease.

In this section, you'll read about many of the major vitamins and minerals. And you will learn about some studies that confirm the health benefit of adding them to your diet. But you will also see a list of foods that are the richest source of each of these nutrients. Whether you supplement or not, make sure you are regularly choosing foods with the highest possible nutrient content.

VITAMIN A

He hadn't named it, but Hippocrates knew about this vitamin hundreds of years before the birth of Christ. He had discovered that eating animal liver was a treatment for night blindness, now known to be caused by a lack of vitamin A.

Vitamin A is important for any passages in your body that open to the outside world—eyes, lungs, bladder, kidneys, and skin. The skin can become dry and scaly, and feel like coarse sandpaper if there is a deficiency (many expensive facial lotions contain vitamin A). Goosebumps on the backs of the upper arms can indicate a deficiency.

Hair-like fibers called *cilia* in the respiratory tract "wave" in a constant motion to keep bacteria off the membrane surfaces. When there is a lack of vitamin A, these fibers lose their wave-like movement, giving the bacteria or virus a foothold. To keep sinus trouble, sore throat, and respiratory infections at bay, make sure you and your family are eating plenty of vitamin A-rich foods.

Beta-carotene is known as vegetable vitamin A because it converts in the body to vitamin A. When food or supplements containing beta-carotene are consumed, the beta-carotene is converted in to vitamin A in the liver.

GETTING VITAMIN A IN YOUR DIET

Include sweet potatoes, carrots, mangos, spinach, dark leafy-green vegetables, cantaloupe, apricots, milk, egg yolks, and mozzarella cheese in the diet.

- Bake sweet potatoes in place of white potatoes. Serve just as you would a regular potato.

- Add one carrot to any fresh juice you make.

- Put a chunk of sweet potato in a smoothie.

- Replace common, nutrient-deficient iceberg lettuce with dark leafy-green vegetables.

- Buy mangos in season and make them a standard fruit in your diet.

- Vitamin A is lost in storage and food preparation. Eat plenty of vitamin A-rich vegetables uncooked or raw.

Vitamin A-Rich Quick Mango Salsa
1½ cups diced firm ripe mango
¼ cup finely diced red onion
¼ cup minced cilantro
¼ cup chopped green onions
Squeeze of lime

- Chop ingredients, mix, and add lime juice. Refrigerate. Serve with fish or chicken.

Vitamin A-Rich Grecian Greens
½ cup kale
1 cup collard greens
½ cup fresh spinach leaves
1 medium garlic clove, diced
½ cup fresh mushrooms, sliced
½ a medium onion, chopped
1 tablespoon butter or olive oil

- Sauté garlic and onion in oil until soft. Add the chopped greens, cover, and lightly sauté for 1 minute. Remove from heat. Garnish with freshly chopped red peppers and parsley.

VITAMIN C

One of the most important vitamins is vitamin C, which prevents scurvy. Scurvy, a disease that affects connective tissue, has been recognized for centuries. Vitamin C is important for maintaining body collagen; helps heal wounds, scars, and fractures; and strengthens blood vessels while giving resistance to infections.

Eighteenth century sailors died more frequently from scurvy than were killed in battle or lost at sea. They had classic vitamin C deficiency signs: bleeding gums, easy bruising, slow healing, nosebleeds, swollen joints, and poor digestion.

Scientists say studies now show that a vitamin C deficiency can severely damage the testes in men, leading to a sperm deficiency and infertility. According to Dr. William A. Harris, M.D., a professor of obstetrics and gynecology at the University of Texas Medical Branch in Galveston:

Building up the body's supply of vitamin C can restore fertility. Dr. Harris gave infertile men 1,000-milligrams of vitamin C a day for sixty days, and the results were startling: sperm were 30 percent more active, the percent of abnormal sperm dropped, and all were able to impregnate their wives at the end of the two-month trial. None of the controls—men not getting vitamin C—were able to do so.

Dr. Harris and colleagues conducted another test to determine how much vitamin C was needed to be effective. Their conclusion: 1,000-milligrams worked faster, but after a couple of weeks, the lower 200-milligram dose they tested was just as effective at bringing sperm count up to fertile quality.[200]

GETTING VITAMIN C IN YOUR DIET

- Eat citrus fruits, strawberries, peppers, cantaloupe, broccoli, kiwi fruit, and alfalfa sprouts.

- Finely dice red peppers and put on your sandwich.

- Add alfalfa sprouts to your salads or sandwiches.

- Keep frozen strawberries on hand and add them to smoothies.

VITAMIN D

You can get vitamin D in your food or by exposure to sunlight. It is called the "sunshine" vitamin because the action of the sun's ultraviolet rays activates a form of cholesterol that is present in the skin and converts to vitamin D.

The textbook deficiency sign is soft bones (rickets), but a lack can also cause muscular numbness, tingling, and spasms. Good food sources are fish liver oils, milk, egg yolk, sprouted seeds, wheatgrass juice, and mushrooms. Most of the body's need for vitamin D can be met by sufficient exposure to sunlight and from small amounts in food. Air pollution, clouds, window glass, and clothing can inhibit absorption.

VITAMIN E

Vitamin E is an antioxidant, which means it stops oxidation (rusting) in the body. It helps prevent saturated fats from breaking down and combining with other substances that may cause internal damage. Vitamin E is also protective of red blood cells and inhibits coagulation and clotting of the blood. Because vitamin E is really a complex of several different co-factors (tocopherol + tocotrienals), your best source is vitamin E-rich foods.

Deficiency signs include rupture of red blood cells, muscular wasting, and abnormal fat deposits in muscles.

Sources of vitamin E include nuts, legumes, seeds, flax, fresh wheat germ (no older than three days; older, rancid germ contains no vitamin E), eggs, cold-pressed oils, dark leafy-green vegetables, sweet potatoes, and molasses.

GETTING VITAMIN E IN YOUR DIET

Sprinkle raw nuts on your salads for a salad "crunchie."

- Sunflower, sesame, and pumpkin seeds are great for snacking or as a topping to casseroles.

  Vitamin E-Rich Southern Sweet Potato Luncheon Salad

  Prepare a bed of leafy greens for salad, including choices such as kale, romaine, spinach, collards, and parsley. Peel and slice one small raw sweet potato into shoestring slices. Cut one boiled egg into six wedges. Arrange the sweet potato slices and egg wedges on the greens. Sprinkle with 1 tablespoon crushed walnuts. Serve with a dressing of cold-pressed almond oil and raw apple cider vinegar. Season to taste.

RODNEY'S VITAMIN E STORY

"GUESS WHAT? RODNEY'S WARTS ARE GONE!"

Gloria came into the Tahoma Clinic to try the newest weight loss plan I was offering based on the best-selling book *Enter the Zone* by Barry Sears, PhD. In tow was her five-year-old son, Rodney, whom she had just picked up from kindergarten. Rodney was quite the gentleman and practiced his coloring while his mother and I completed her plan.

I noticed that Rodney had warts all over both hands. He even had warts growing on top of warts! Quite a sight! They covered both hands but were particularly bad on his thumbs.

I asked Gloria about the warts. "They just came on suddenly last year. We've had the doctor burn them off twice, but they just grow back. His classmates make fun of him."

I had read that there were some relatively simple and safe natural remedies that had been shown to get rid of warts. One of these remedies was vitamin E oil, straight and strong, applied to them several times throughout the day. I mentioned this vitamin E remedy to Gloria as she and Rodney were leaving my office.

Several weeks later I had a call from Gloria. She was elated! "Guess what? Rodney's warts are gone! It's just a miracle!"

I asked her what she had done.

"I tried the vitamin E. We applied it several times a day faithfully. Nothing happened for a couple weeks, then magic! They began to disappear until his little hands were completely clear!"

—

So here is a simple example of just how powerful natural remedies can be. Vitamin E is just one of many natural remedies that are said to get rid of warts.

③④ The Vitamin B Complex

The vitamin B family helps to maintain healthy nerves in addition to numerous other functions. As a general rule of thumb, a deficiency of one often indicates a deficiency of another because all the B vitamins work as a team. Following is a description of each of the B vitamins.

VITAMIN B-1 (THIAMINE)

Thiamine is called B-1 because it was the first B vitamin to be isolated in 1927. It has been referred to as the morale or nerve vitamin since it is needed for a healthy mental attitude. It has been used in the treatment of alcoholism.

Thiamine is a part of the germ and bran of wheat and the husk of rice—the portion of all grains that is routinely milled out, giving the grain a lighter color and finer texture. White-flour products are notoriously thiamine-deficient.

Foods rich in thiamine are sunflower seeds, whole-grains, tuna, black beans, green peas, pinto beans, lentils, bananas, and corn.

GETTING THIAMINE IN YOUR DIET

- Buy bananas that are marked down because they are speckled. Peel and cut in chunks. Freeze to use in smoothies.

- Buy a dehydrator and dehydrate green peas to use as salad crunchies.

- Add sunflower seeds to tuna or chicken salad.
  Vitamin B-1 Rich Black Bean Picnic Salad

1 can black beans, drained and rinsed

1 small onion, chopped

1 red pepper, chopped

1 cup frozen corn, thawed

4 tablespoons sunflower seeds

- Mix all ingredients. Add a vinegar and oil or Italian dressing.

RIBOFLAVIN (VITAMIN B-2)

In the early 1940s, this vitamin was made widely available because of the enrichment program which added synthetic B-2 back to processed foods. The newly immerging white-flour products had been stripped! The enrichment program makes a vitamin B-2 deficiency unusual, but anyone who has dieted excessively, has food idiosyncrasies, or has long-standing bad eating habits (a diet built on sugar, for example) can become deficient.

Some signs of deficiency are dandruff, cracks and sores at corners of the mouth, flaky skin, a sore tongue, and light sensitivity. Excessive use of alcohol, contraceptives, or too strenuous of exercise can deplete riboflavin.

GETTING RIBOFLAVIN IN YOUR DIET

- These foods are good sources: brewer's or nutritional yeast, brown rice, cheese, egg yolks, fish, legumes, nuts, liver, peas, whole grains, and yogurt.

- Get rid of the white rice and replace it with brown rice. If you learn to cook brown rice properly, you will enjoy it as much or more than white rice.

- Keep nutritional yeast on hand, and use it like Parmesan cheese, sprinkling it on hot popcorn, garlic bread, etc. Try stirring a spoonful into a stir-fry or a pasta dish. Nutritional yeast can be found in the bulk or supplement section of your health food store. You'll find nutritional yeast flakes or powder.

- Dehydrate peas and use as salad crunchies or in trail mix.

- Snack on raw nuts (right out of the shell, not from a can) instead of potato chips or cookies.

NIACIN (B-3)

Niacin is important for a properly functioning nervous system. It has been used to lower cholesterol and to help prevent a second heart attack.

A common reaction to taking supplemental niacin is what is called a niacin flush—redness, tingling, and a burning sensation throughout the body. It is short-lived and harmless, but alarming. Use of the niacinamide form of B-3 will not result in this niacin flush.

Eating too many refined starches or too much sugar can deplete the body's supply of niacin. Deficiencies include muscle weakness, fatigue, indigestion, skin eruptions, canker sores, vomiting, insomnia, irritability, tender gums, and nervous disorders.

GETTING NIACIN IN YOUR DIET

- The foods you will want to eat are chicken, tuna, salmon, corn, ground beef, peanuts, potatoes with skins, crimini mushrooms, lean meats, brewer's yeast, and rice bran.

- Include brown rice in your diet.

- Keep nutritional yeast in the cupboard and add it to your smoothies, sprinkle on salads and put into casseroles.

Niacin Rich Carolina Corn Salad
> 6 ears corn, husked and cleaned
> 3 large tomatoes, diced
> 1 large onion, diced
> ¼ cup chopped fresh basil
> 2 tablespoons red wine vinegar
> Salt and pepper to taste
> ¼ cup olive oil

- Briefly cook corncobs in salted water. Do not overcook. Drain, cool, and cut kernels off the cob. Toss together the corn, tomatoes, onion, basil, oil, vinegar, salt, and pepper. Chill.

PANTOTHENIC ACID (B-5)

The name of this vitamin comes from a Greek word meaning "from everywhere." Because pantothenic acid is found in most foods, deficiencies of it are not commonly seen in people consuming a nutrient-dense diet. Look at this list of foods rich in pantothenic acid, and ask yourself if you eat any of them regularly: peanuts, whole-grains, beans, almonds, corn, honey, royal jelly, salmon, and legumes. Deficiency signs are fatigue, depression, adrenal exhaustion and sleep disturbances.

GETTING PANTOTHENIC ACID IN YOUR DIET

- Get off white bread and pastas; switch to whole-grain varieties. Pasta products made from whole-grains are available in natural food stores.

- Learn to cook beans of all kinds. They are very cheap and high in protein. Always soak beans prior to cooking (per package directions) to avoid intestinal gas.

- Use honey instead of white sugar.

- Get wild salmon in the diet frequently, up to twice a week if you are not vegan.

Bee Sweet Carmel Corn

8 to 10 cups of popped corn, add:

1 cup of your favorite nuts

- In a pan, melt 2 tablespoons butter or olive oil, ½ cup honey, ½ cup blackstrap molasses. Stir in popcorn and nuts until totally coated. To crisp, place on a cookie sheet, and bake at a very low temperature—175 degrees for 20 to 30 minutes.

PYRIDOXINE (B-6)

If you have greasy dermatitis around your eyes and eyebrows, or at the corners of the mouth, it could indicate a deficiency of the vitamin called pyridoxine, and eating more B-6-rich foods is in order. Pyridoxine is also associated with relief of menstrual symptoms, including headaches, edema, bloating, depression, and irritability. If you buy a PMS formula at a health food store, it will likely contain vitamin B-6, among other key ingredients. B-6 is also associated with a reduced risk of heart disease.

GETTING PYRIDOXINE IN YOUR DIET

- Rich food sources are whole-grains, turnip greens, salmon, beans, seeds, blackstrap molasses, dark green and leafy vegetables and meat. Processed foods have had most of the pyridoxine removed. If you eat whole food, you will sidestep this problem.

- Have you ever tried turnip greens? If you are from the south, I'll bet you have! Lightly steam them, season well, and serve with a little olive oil or butter and a dash of apple cider vinegar on top.

- Rather than always serving the kids "noodle soups," buy healthy bean soups in a natural food store.

- Sprinkle sesame seeds or sunflower seeds on salads or sandwiches.

- Get a juicer; add a variety of dark leafy-green vegetables to the juice. See *www.gethealthyamerica.biz* for a juicer and a greens product.

Vitamin B-6 Rich Molasses Toddy

For an afternoon pick-me-up beverage, in eight ounces of hot water, stir in 2–3 teaspoons of blackstrap molasses, a few drops of pure vanilla, and 1 teaspoon of milk or milk alternative (like soy, almond, or rice milks). Sprinkle with ground cinnamon, or garnish with a cinnamon stick.

FOLIC ACID

This important B vitamin derives is name from the Latin folium, which means "foliage or leaf." It is so named because it was first isolated from spinach and was known to be abundant in dark green, leafy plants. There is a plethora of information these days about the importance of folic acid to prevent birth defects. It is one of the nutrients most often deficient in our diets.

The Medical Research Council in Britain studied 1,817 women who had previously had a child with neural tube defects (NTD) to see if they could lower the recurrence rate with multivitamins or folate (4 milligrams daily). These women were compared with 1,195 who had children without NTD. Significant protective effect was observed in the groups that received folic acid compared with the groups that did not.[201]

GETTING FOLIC ACID IN YOUR DIET

- These foods are good sources: green and leafy vegetables, liver, root vegetables, whole-grains, asparagus, beef, dates, bran, cheese, and brewer's yeast.

- Do you ever eat root vegetables? Bake yams and sweet potatoes occasionally rather than a plain potato; mash parsnips or turnips like potatoes; steam beets; and try all of these raw and cut-up, served with vegetable dip (rather than chips).

- Give up common iceberg lettuce in favor of dark, leafy greens. Wash and store so you will have them ready for salad.

- Eat asparagus in season. It's yummy raw or as part of a salad.

CYANOCOBALAMIN (B-12)

This is the last of the B-complex vitamins discovered in 1948. Every cell in the body depends upon B-12. All B-12 is manufactured by microorganisms that normally reside in the intestines, so it is not typically found in fruits and vegetables. However, some fermented foods and other foods contain small amounts.

Vegetarians and vegans (vegetarians may eat dairy products; vegans eat no animal products or anything, like cheese, made from an animal) are consistently advised to make sure they are getting enough B-12 in their diet because it is typically found in meat, dairy, and egg. Many vegans and vegetarians fulfill their needs by consuming a greens product that contains spirulina. For an excellent greens product, see *www.gethealthyamerica.biz.*

Signs of deficiency are fatigue, nervousness, and dizziness.

GETTING B-12 IN YOUR DIET

- These foods are good sources: meat, fish, eggs, dairy, fermented soybean products, vegetable burger mixes, textured vegetable protein, sprouts, nuts, bananas, and alfalfa.

- Add sprouts of all sorts to your food (see sprouting section).

- If you are vegetarian, there are many fermented soy products available in natural foods stores—miso, tempeh, and sea vegetables are examples. Generally, if you are a vegetarian, it is advisable to supplement with B-12.

B-12 Rich Alfalfa Nectar

To 1 quart of hot water, add 1 tablespoon alfalfa leaves. Steep a few moments. Sweeten with honey or Stevia herbal sweetener, if desired.

PANGAMIC ACID (B-15)

Pangamic acid is not widely recognized and often not recognized as a vitamin. It is important for increasing oxygen in the blood and improving circulation. Food sources are sesame seeds, sunflower seeds, and black walnuts.

BIOTIN

Biotin keeps hair, skin, and glands healthy. Consuming large amounts of antibiotics causes a deficiency of this vitamin.[202] A deficiency of biotin can result in dry skin, lack of energy, dermatitis, gray skin color, and baldness. Food sources are egg yolks, beef liver, unpolished rice, nutritional yeast, cauliflower, and mushrooms.

CHOLINE & INOSITOL

Choline and Inositol are in the vitamin B complex. These help with fat metabolism, hair growth, and nerve function. Food sources are eggs, turnips, nuts, soybeans, peanuts, and beef.

THE MINERALS

③⑤ Calcium to Zinc

Minerals are naturally occurring elements found in the earth that all living cells require. Minerals work like coenzymes, which means they help enzymes in the body in carrying out all of the daily activities as efficiently as possible.

Minerals are categorized into two groups: macrominerals and trace minerals. Marcominerals are needed in larger amounts and include calcium, magnesium, sodium, potassium, and phosphorus. Trace minerals are required in very small amounts but are absolutely essential to your health. These include boron, chromium, copper, germanium, iodine, iron, manganese, molybdenum, selenium, silicon, sulfur, vanadium, and zinc.[203] In this section, we will discuss a few of the most commonly known minerals.

CALCIUM

Calcium is needed for strong bones and teeth, regular heartbeat, and nerve health. It is used to keep the gums healthy and to prevent muscle cramping and osteoporosis. Common deficiency signs are cavities, muscle cramps, arthritis, and nervousness.

GETTING CALCIUM IN YOUR DIET

- You'll want to eat salmon (fresh or canned with bones), sesame seeds, sardines, dark leafy-green vegetables, asparagus, dairy foods, collards, watercress, oats, prunes, figs, filberts, paprika, tofu, yogurt, and almonds.

- When I was a flight attendant in years gone by, when airline food was really good, we made a beautiful salad in first class. It was simply fresh watercress with a dressing of sour cream, mixed with a dab of horseradish. That was it! We added a little salt and freshly ground pepper. Look for fresh watercress in your store and give it a try!

- Lightly sauté collard greens in a little olive oil or butter with fresh, diced garlic. Serve with chopped filberts on top.

MAGNESIUM

Magnesium is a tireless worker that is involved in energy production and nerve and muscle impulses. It also protects against artery damage. A deficiency in your diet can lead to constipation (milk of magnesia is for constipation), confusion, heart problems, depression, insomnia and nervous disorders.

GETTING MAGNESIUM IN YOUR DIET

- You will need to add some of these foods to your diet: apples, almonds, cashews, soybeans, spinach, nuts, oatmeal, potato, and dark leafy-green vegetables. Whole-wheat—not white flour—is a good source. The Standard American Diet, highly refined, is notoriously deficient in magnesium-rich foods.

- Stop eating white-flour products (see section on whole grains).

- Have oatmeal with chopped almonds and cashews occasionally for breakfast.

Magnesium Rich Applesauce with a Punch

2 cups raw apples

½ cup plain yogurt

½ cup raisins

½ cup chopped fresh coconut

¼ cup wheat germ or oat bran

½ lemon

1–2 tablespoons honey

- Blend chopped apples with enough water to make a medium-firm sauce. Squeeze in the juice of ½ a lemon to keep the apples from turning brown. Add 1 to 2 tablespoons honey, if desired. Blend. Stir in remaining ingredients. Chill and serve garnished with chopped walnuts or pecans.

MANGANESE

Manganese deficiency can affect glucose/sugar metabolism. Low levels are also associated with atherosclerosis.

Dr. Jeanne Freeland-Graves from the University of Texas explains the importance of manganese for bones. Animals low in manganese get severe osteoporosis. In one study, she found that osteoporotic women had one third less manganese in their blood than healthy women.

When these women were given manganese, their bodies absorbed about twice as much, showing that they needed it. Dr. Freeland-Graves says that when we want to up a woman's manganese in the diet, we tell women to eat pineapple and drink pineapple juice. [204]

Deficiencies include atherosclerosis, eye and hearing problems, and improper blood sugar regulation.

GETTING MANGANESE IN YOUR DIET

- Sources are avocados, pineapple, whole grains, egg yolks, nuts, seeds, and green vegetables.

- Buy fresh pineapple. If it seems expensive, consider that the average serving is no more costly than one can of soda.

- Add sliced avocado to sandwiches, salads, and smoothies.

  Manganese Rich Pineapple Splash Smoothie
  ½ orange
  ½ cup fresh pineapple
  ½ frozen banana
  ½ cup orange juice
  Ice as desired

- Mix all ingredients in a blender until smooth. You may add your favorite protein powder. See *www.gethealthyamerica.biz* for a heavy-duty blender.

POTASSIUM

The mineral potassium, along with sodium, helps regulate the body's water balance. Potassium is very important for proper heartbeat and helps regulate nerve impulses. Some studies say that having enough potassium in your diet can help prevent strokes.

GETTING POTASSIUM IN YOUR DIET

- These foods are good sources: all vegetables, oranges, whole-grains, sunflower seeds, potatoes (especially skins), spinach, blackstrap molasses, tomato juice, sardines, and bananas.

- Sprinkle sunflower seeds on salads, sandwiches, and casseroles.

- Roll bananas in chopped sunflower seeds. Freeze on popsicle sticks for snacks.

- Eat the skin of your baked potato.

- Try blackstrap molasses rather than sugar to sweeten your herbal tea.

Peppy Potassium Pleaser
1 carrot
½ cup raw spinach
1 fresh tomato
1 handful of parsley
1 small garlic clove

- Put ingredients through a juicer. Serve over ice, with a sprig of parsley and a lemon wedge. Season to taste.

SELENIUM

Selenium is a mineral that works in your body as an antioxidant. Simply put, an antioxidant keeps you from rusting on the inside. Selenium protects your body and immune system by preventing the formation of the *free radicals* that cause this rusting process.

Here is a study that might interest men:

The International Journal of Cancer found that among 445 U.S. men, high blood concentrations of selenium appeared to reduce by 30 percent the risk that a man would develop prostate cancer. Selenium is a constituent of the enzyme glutathione peroxidase, one of the body's more potent antioxidants. Such agents have the ability to quash biologically damaging reactions triggered within the body by any of a host of naturally produced chemicals called oxidants. Because oxidant damage has been linked with many cancers, some scientists have suspected that any anticancer benefit from selenium probably would trace to its antioxidant contribution."[205]

Deficiency signs include heart disease and joint problems. Some studies have associated deficiency states with high cholesterol and cancer. These foods are good dietary additions: Brazil nuts (highest source; eat in moderation), tuna, beef, cod, lamb, barley, mushrooms, broccoli, onions, and garlic.

GETTING SELENIUM IN YOUR DIET

- Try eating chopped Brazil nuts (in moderation—only 1–2 daily) instead of salted, oiled peanuts.

- Sauté mushrooms in olive oil with finely chopped garlic and onions for a vegetable alternative.

ZINC

Zinc is a prostate-friendly mineral needed for a healthy reproductive system. When you have a cut or wound, zinc will be involved in healing. This mineral is also important to fight off colds and the flu. The most common cause of zinc deficiency is an unbalanced diet.

Deficiency signs include loss of taste and/or smell, acne, delayed sexual maturation, fatigue, hair loss, susceptibility to infection, colds, and slow wound healing.

GETTING ZINC IN YOUR DIET

- Good sources are nutritional yeast, kelp, egg yolks, fish, legumes, peas, pumpkin seeds, poultry, sardines, mushrooms, and parsley.

- There are some very good canned bean soups in the natural food section of your store. Keep these on hand for quick lunches.

Zinc Rich Mushroom Salad

Wash and thinly slice one cup of fresh mushrooms. Finely dice one fresh garlic clove, and mix with mushrooms. Stir in ¾ cup peas. Bind together with a little sour cream or plain yogurt. Place a scoop of the salad on a bed of greens, and sprinkle with one-tablespoon pumpkin seeds. Serve as a side dish to lean turkey patties or baked chicken. Hulled pumpkin seeds are mild and delicious. They are available in natural food stores.

A HISTORIC LOOK AT NUTRITION

3 6 Elizabeth Baker's History Lesson

(Recorded at a Get Healthy, America! Seminar, Tampa, 2003)

Ron: Elizabeth, if you will come to the microphone, we'll let the audience begin with questions. Why don't you start by talking about Dr. Weston Price's work? Many of the people in our audience have seen his video this weekend. But for the benefit of those who haven't…

Elizabeth: Okay. I think that history will remember Dr. Price's work as pivotal in the course of human nutrition. It was in the 1930s that Dr. Price, a dentist, and his wife began a ten-year journey of worldwide travels. They were studying remote cultures where the people lived entirely on indigenous foods.

Audience: What do you mean by indigenous?

Elizabeth: Well, I suppose you could say homegrown. The common denominator among all the people was they ate the foods their ancestors had eaten for generations. They had never been introduced to, eaten, or for that matter even seen processed foods—sugar and refined white flour, canned foods, pasteurized milk, packaged dinners, and the rest.

Ron: Do you recall where they traveled over the ten years?

Elizabeth: They visited remote Swiss villages, the Eskimos in Alaska, traditional American Indians, African tribes, and Australian Aborigines. Dr. Prices' studies were considered unique in history because the people hadn't had any contact with civilization and so called "civilized foods." If you tried to recreate the study today, it would be impossible because modern civilization has reached almost every corner of the world.

Audience: I have his book, isn't it called *Nutrition and Physical Degeneration?*

Elizabeth: Yes.

Audience: I haven't read it, but it sure has some amazing photos in it!

Ron: That's right. Actually, Dr. Price took thousands of photos of teeth, mouths, and physical stature. His photos demonstrate that people who stray from their traditional diets have narrowed jaws, crowded and decayed teeth, and general body degeneration.

Elizabeth: Yes, and his photos show that down through the generations, cultures that stay with their native foods have children with healthy, broad smiles and healthy teeth. If they begin eating modern foods—or as he called them, the foods of commerce—become a part of the diet, the children then born begin to have dental problems and are susceptible to infectious and chronic disease, even birth defects!

Audience: I saw the video here at the seminar yesterday. I thought it was interesting that the diets of the healthy cultures were diverse. Everything from heavy meat eaters to complete vegetarians, and everything in between—some cooked and some raw foods.

Elizabeth: Yes, but all the foods were the native, traditional foods eaten by their ancestors. No foods of civilization as he called them.

Ron: Let's move on to the Pottenger cat studies in the 1940s.

Elizabeth: Okay. It was in the 1940s that Dr. Frances Pottenger did extensive food studies on cats. He studied hundreds of cats over ten years, which he divided into three groups. The first group was fed a wholesome raw food diet—raw meats and milk. The second group got partly-cooked and partly-raw food. And the poor third group was given all cooked foods and highly-sugared condensed milk or pasteurized milk. Does anyone in the audience remember this study?

Audience: Yes. I am just old enough to remember. Wasn't the story covered in the newspapers of the day? And, didn't the third group become sick?

Elizabeth: Yes, and very sick! The cats were nervous, neurotic, had soft bones and bad temperaments. They were unable to reproduce after the third generation. The cooked foods they lived on caused them to have thick mucous membranes, allergy symptoms, respiratory infections, even arthritis. Pottenger found the same things happened to his human patients when they ate a processed, cooked, nutrient-devoid diet. Again, as in Dr. Price's work, when humans—or animals—move away from their native diets, they begin to degenerate.

Ron: Time is running short, so let's move on to the fiber studies by Denis Burkitt.

Elizabeth: Well that was in the 1970s. In his travels, he found that native African cultures didn't have the diseases common to Western cultures—heart attacks, cancer, high blood pressure, obesity, diabetes, constipation, even gallstones.

Audience: So why don't these cultures have our diseases?

Elizabeth: His studies pinpointed their high-fiber diet and low intake of refined carbohydrates. Dr. Burkitt also found there was a correlation between the emergence of these diseases in the United States and England following the introduction of a new milling technique (after 1890) that removed fiber from whole-grain flour to produce white flour. There is no fiber in white flour.

Audience: That's interesting. I understand what fiber has to do with constipation but not with heart problems and cancer.

Elizabeth: Dr. Burkitt found that civilized people eating fiber-less, refined foods, forgive me, had fewer bowel movements. They retained food up to one week as compared to the Africans who eliminated up to three times a day. A toxic condition existed in the bodies of the civilized people's diet. He explains the details in his work.

Ron: Well, we are just about out of time. Can you briefly discuss the work of Otto Schaefer, M.D.

Elizabeth: Yes. Otto Schaeffer's work was in the late 1960s. He spent decades of his medical career in northern Canada—with the Inuit peoples. He traveled by dogsled and stayed in igloos in remote Inuit camps treating sick people and documenting their health problems. His research is well established in medical literature. Like the other researchers we've discussed, he tracked Greenland and Alaskan Eskimos as they moved into a new modern life. By living with these peoples and studying trading post records, he found that by the mid-1940s, there were dramatic changes in their lives. They were eating and working at the emerging military bases and basically living on the foods of commerce, as Dr. Price would put it. Their diets became rich in processed foods, chocolates, and sugary soda pop—things they had never eaten before. There was a quite sudden rise in the diseases of civilization—diabetes, heart problems, and gallbladder surgery. And

279

acne in the teenagers. The message is clear—stay with whole, natural foods and don't eat the processed junk of this generation; that is, assuming you want good health and a long life.

Ron: Thanks, Elizabeth. What a wealth of information you've given us to think about. I suppose the question we all need to consider is, do our food practices today cause similar changes in our modern society? Your historic information certainly gives us cause to pause and think.

For more information on these topics, go to *www.gethealthyamerica.biz.*

③⑦ Elizabeth Baker Tells Her Cancer Story

(As recorded in private journals of Elizabeth Baker, and left to me as a precious gift after her death. The story was written on an old typewriter and the pages had become yellowed with age.)

"My cancer story began, I have no doubt, in 1952, when I was given the maximum dosage of the "miracle" antibiotic, Chloromycetin, for pneumonia. It truly changed my life. I recovered in record time, but I continued to run a low-grade temperature for a year and a half.

From then on I was very susceptible to colds and flu. I ran a temperature for years afterwards with energy levels so low I was unable to do any physical work or even walk a block. Between such periods, which represented half of the time, I had only fair energy and little endurance.

Not until some ten years after taking the Chloromycetin did I learn that it could and in most cases did destroy bone marrow where the white "defense" cells are made. This knowledge at least answered the nagging question as to why my white count in every blood test showed 20% of normal.

From the time of the Chloromycetin episode, my health began to go down until 1977 when cancer was diagnosed. I experienced so many different health problems no one would believe. Eighteen of those twenty-five years I went from one doctor to another, to many clinics and laboratories for special tests, landed in several hospitals for surgery I didn't need and special treatments that proved useless or harmful."

TAKING MY HEALTH INTO MY OWN HANDS

In 1970, when my chemist husband realized that certain prescription drugs I was taking were the cause of near-fatal potassium deficiency, he began to encourage and help me take my health care into my own hands.

From then on I struggled for survival day by day, week by week, year by year, through "terminal" Addison's disease, arthritis, colitis, duodenal ulcer, alternate diarrhea and constipation, severe ecological allergies, tic douloureux, hiatal hernia, shingles, osteoporosis, chronic indigestion, bursitis and bronchitis, to mention a partial list of diseases that wracked my body.

Gradually I conquered most of them including hemorrhoids and painful, bleeding intestinal polyps I nearly had removed by surgery. Despite freedom from many of these ills that the conventional medical profession considers incurable or untreatable without surgery and drugs, I still had to deal with anemia.

Then, when I passed old, black, coagulated blood clots, I knew something ominous was happening. Because I had been for several years on an all-natural, 50% raw diet, with all allergy-causing foods eliminated, I felt I would never have cancer. I was wrong. After learning I had a malignant tumor in the ascending colon (a dull pain had plagued me for two years), I realized that I had had it for a long time. As it was a slow-growing kind, my nutritionist physician said it had probably started between fifteen and twenty years before, maybe even longer. I also had for years small skin cancers on my face and a large one on the back of my hand.

With the positive verdict of cancer of the ascending colon, the doctors immediately set plans in motion for taking care of the cancer. The procedure was routine. My case, according to them, was just another of the type they dealt with every day. The surgery they began to discuss would probably result in a colostomy. Then there would be chemotherapy and radiation. How many months or years I had left would have to be determined as I "progressed."

HOW NARROW THE PATH OF THE DRASTIC TREATMENT

I was shocked at how established, how automated, how categorized, how narrow was the path of the drastic, destroying treatment. I would almost be like a thing on the conveyer belt of an assembly line. Yet I was an individual, different as each patient is different from every other one. No two are ever alike in any way for a multitude of reasons.

I had already learned there were many alternate therapies for diseases. I had already proven to myself with God's constant guidance and my own efforts, my body could conquer them. God gave us a marvelous creation in the form of our bodies. It was made to self-heal if treated the way He intended.

I thought of the Bible that teaches us how to nourish it the way He originally intended. "I gave every seed-bearing plant on the face of the whole earth and every tree that has fruit with seed in it. They will be yours for food" (Genesis 1:29, NIV). And "...the tree of life bearing twelve crops of fruit, yielding its fruit every month—and leaves—for the healing of the nations" (Revelation 22:2, NIV).

Politely, quietly, I listened to the plans for the dreadful ordeal the doctors laid out for me. I left without saying a word, not because I was overwhelmed for my own welfare, but because I saw a veritable slow-death running full speed in the hands of determined physicians whose minds were closed to the wishes of the patient and the natural, painless, constructive ways of healing God taught us to employ.

In the fresh air outside the hospital clinic, I made my decision for I was sure God was looking down on me with great understanding.

Jesus stood by me in love and compassion. His words rang like clear bells in my mind. "I will never leave thee." And the indwelling of the Holy Spirit filled me with peace and the assurance of recovery. I was joyous. I was radiant. I knew the direction I would not take: the direction that led to the "cut, poison, burn" modalities.

I WAS PREPARED FOR MY DECISION

Years of nutrition study had prepared me for the decision. I recalled reading the booklet of Christine Nolfi, M.D., of Denmark. She cured herself of breast cancer by an all-raw diet. If she could, I could, I told myself. I also had read Ann Wigmore's *Be Your Own Doctor,* which bolstered my confidence.

At that time my husband, Elton, was away for two weeks. I had decided to stay home, consult an internist about the pain in my side, then do some shopping for our October trip to Australia with the International College of Applied Nutrition.

When I met my returning dear one at the airport, we were so caught up in happiness on seeing each other and chatting about his successful trip, I could not bring myself to tell him about the verdict of cancer. As the hours spun by in joy and sharing, I decided not to tell him. There was no reason to. Although my health was not vigorous, it was good enough to withstand the mild rigors of today's travel. Besides, he might have cancelled our reservations in an effort to protect me had he known. He would be greatly disappointed. I didn't want that.

By touring Australia and New Zealand in their spring, we would find an abundance of fresh fruit and vegetables for my raw diet. We did, and I enjoyed the trip immensely, benefiting from it in many ways.

WHY A RAW DIET?

Why a raw diet? Because 30% to 85% of the nutrition in natural foods is destroyed in cooking. That is an average of 50% loss. I knew a cancer patient could not afford to eat anything that is not health giving if he or she wanted to get well.

There are two more reasons I should mention. Cancer cells proliferate only where there is not enough oxygen for cells to be healthy. Give the area and the whole body optimal oxygen and the cancer can't proliferate. Raw foods contain an abundance of oxygen. In cooked foods, oxygen is destroyed. This is a powerful fact. A truth. Jesus said, "Ye shall know the truth and the truth shall make ye free." I knew someday I would be free of cancer if I learned to use the patience and persistence God gave me.

The other reason for eating only living (raw) foods is they give more energy. They contain "all" the nutrients for energy intact, unaltered. They digest so easily only 10% of one's total energy is used.

Conventional, mostly cooked and processed foods take 30% of total energy for digestion. That is a 20% more energy expenditure than for raw food digestion. This means anyone on an all-raw diet has at least 20% more energy than the average person not on it. Actually, processed foods are full of toxic additives that take their toll on bodily energy. Add to that reduced body function efficiency (I could go on), we find even more than a 20% bonus in energy for the raw-food eating person. It's more like 50% more energy for the raw food eater than the average eater.

For me, there was every reason for an all-raw diet and none against. Not one. Besides, I much preferred the delicious, natural taste.

My cancer battle was not the toughest one I ever fought but it was the longest—two years and two months. My first great skirmish was discovering I had to eat more than just the fruits and vegetables and few seeds and nuts the ten or twelve raw-food books advocated. Hunger, the powerful motivator, spurred me on to learn of all the raw foods available, how to sprout every kind of edible seed I could buy, then figure out ways I could prepare them to satisfy my taste, cravings, and weight needs.

THE UNCOOK BOOK

It didn't take long to do that. But writing it in a form acceptable for publication that would answer the many questions audiences, classes, and counselees would ask, took nearly a year. That publication, *The Uncook Book*, is, in essence, the account of the way I conquered cancer: the foods, the supplements, the green drinks containing dandelion and comfrey, the wheatgrass juice, the how-tos and don'ts, and the whys.

It does not say anything about exercises, which were a daily part of my recovery program. That is in *Bandwagon to Health*, the book that followed. But neither tells the final chapter of my cancer battle story, a skirmish that nearly ended in tragedy, the tragedy of failure, of surgery, chemotherapy, and radiation.

It was early March 1979, and we were returning from Mexico on planes that missed connections. We endured trying situations not expected, fatigue, and finally unusually raw cold upon returning to our home on the Puget Sound in Seattle. My low immune system could not cope with the severe bronchial pneumonia I sank into. With intravenous vitamin C for two weeks in a hospital, I was up again, but barely so.

The usual low-grade temperature following a respiratory infection kept me so throttled I was more down than up. In May, realizing I was not progressing, I went for three weeks to a living foods health resort I had been to before (the Hippocrates Institute). I left after two weeks to go home to bed. I was ill.

Summer passed quickly because I was writing all the time (in bed) on *The Uncook Book*. But by mid-August I realized I needed help. Because of a real obstruction in the lower right side of my colon, my digestive system was hardly functioning.

As I was suffering a peculiar allergy, I went to see my internationally known allergist. She took one look at me and demanded, "Have you got cancer? You are ashy white." She knew and wanted to scare me into action.

THAT'S A SKIN CANCER!

I told her of the diagnosis two years before and my other baffling problems. She interrupted me to take the bandage off my hand. "That's a skin cancer," she said, giving the dime-size lesion a long, scary name. "That's a deep one. How long has it been there?" I told her seven years. "Have it removed before it involves the tendons any more," she scolded. I smiled but thought a frown. Surgery might remove it, but it would mutilate my hand, leave vast scar tissue, and probably permanently cripple my fingers.

The good lady continued, "I want you to go to University Hospital and get a Carcenoembryonic Antigen Test tomorrow." She wrote out the order as soon as she finished taking care of my allergy and dismissed me with a short, "I'll call you."

A week later to the day she called me. "You're as high as you can be on the positive side of the CEA test," she declared. I felt sure she was trying to push me to what she felt was the logical, the safe, sane, physical, visual approach to handling cancer.

Conventional doctors have to "see" their cases by X-ray, laser, fluoroscope, special lights, or an incision that lays open the innards. They find it increasingly difficult to believe the invisible healing God has for us for the asking. I asked her what she would suggest I do. Her answer was quick and sure: "Find the best possible colon-cancer surgeon and have that tumor out immediately." I asked another question or two to avoid any comment, thanked her, and hung up.

"Oh Lord, my precious Lord," I prayed, "You'll have to tell me again what to do. Do you really not want me to have surgery? I'm all out of ideas. I've come to the end of my resources. Shall I have surgery?"

It was about 10:30 a.m. and I lay exhausted and in limbo: physically, spiritually, and mentally. Weakness and the sharp pains of indigestion enveloped me. Had I missed God's will for me? Was I at the end of my narrow road full of rocks, chuckholes, and ominous overhanging cliffs?

THE VALLEY OF THE SHADOW OF DEATH

Was I not going to make it through the valley of the shadow of death? I prayed fervently but went to sleep before I finished. When I awoke at 1:00 p.m., Elton was standing over me with a small dish of fresh peaches he had pureed in the blender. When he learned I did not dare add more food to my small undigested breakfast, his face fell. "Maybe you'd better water fast. What do you think?" We discussed it briefly and I agreed, but I dreaded the long, lonely sleeplessness of a fast.

That was Friday morning. The following Tuesday morning I awoke feeling better but so weak Elton had to help me to the bathroom. We had been in touch each day of my water fast with the doctor on the Oregon coast who, six years before, had supervised my eight-day diagnostic water fast that left me well and wise to the allergy-causing foods that had been making me so very ill. When Elton reported to him the morning situation, he agreed with our suggestion to continue on with a juice fast.

We started with two ounces of freshly made apple juice diluted with water and continued with a different kind and increased the amount of freshly extracted juice every three hours. My digestion began to function, and I felt better and progressively had more energy.

The morning of the eighth day of the juice fast, I went to the bathroom for a wonderful elimination. It was huge, of proper consistency, diameter, and color. With it came a large, greenish-gray/blackish, firm, dense mass about 3½ inches long and ¾ of an inch thick. Somehow I knew beyond the shadow of a doubt it was the old, dead tumor. I yelled for Elton to come. Upon seeing it, he was as excited as me. We laughed, and cried, and hugged, and kissed.

MY HEALTH BEGAN TO IMPROVE

From that day on, my health improved, steadily, with no interruptions. I felt so cleansed, so clear-headed, so near to my Maker. The low-grade temperature, which had plagued me since the March pneumonia, faded away. I began to gain energy and weight. By December I felt well. I had finished *The Uncook Book*, sent it off to the publisher, and we were preparing for lecturing in California en route to our winter home in Mexico. I felt great but I had to "know" what the doctors wouldn't believe because they could not see. So, again, I took the CEA test. Afterwards, we drove on to California.

Soon after we arrived, our number two son in Portland called to give us the report of all clear for the CEA test. No cancer. That was wonderful, yet not enough. Needing more assurance, we consulted several alternate-therapy cancer specialists. Two of them had patients who passed their cancerous tumors when the walls of the colon healed and expelled the intruder, the cancer.

A colonic specialist we talked to said she'd had three patients pass their cancers when the colon became healthy. She had preserved one in a sealed jar for private showing. She explained the difference between a dead, un-dissolved, little-shrunken tumor and a rubber-like contained mass of old colon mucous. The tumor was threadlike and black, with wiggly lines all through it, which were the dead blood of the fine veins of the tumor.

Again, we were assured, but again we felt there was one last step in putting to rest the story of my cancer. I had the Dr. Harold Harper test and the Arthur-Amid test. Both showed no sign of cancer. There was still another assurance, an unplanned one. Just before leaving San Diego for Mexico, I took off the Band-Aid, showered, and started to gently dry my hand as I'd had to do for seven years.

But now there was no need to be careful; the cancer was gone. There was no more deep, flaking scab the size of a dime. There was only wonderful, smooth, clean skin with such a tiny scar I could scarcely see it—just enough to keep me reminded and thankful. How beautiful is healing! How great are God and Jesus and the Holy Spirit who saw me through the valley of the shadow of death. [206]

—

Elizabeth lived another thirty-two years in vibrant health, still writing, lecturing, driving and inspiring everyone who met her.

BEGINNING THE JOURNEY

3 8 Detoxification for Optimum Health

Total body detoxification is a natural addition to any health program. An overload of additives, preservatives, stabilizers, artificial colors, rancid fats, sugars, and chemicals of all sorts have become an inevitable consequences of twenty-first century living. When our bodies become too heavily bombarded and poisoned, the normal detoxification pathways cease to work effectively, and the chemicals remain somewhere in the body.

You can help rid your body of toxins at the cellular level by drinking plenty of pure water, having regular bowel movements, deeply inhaling clean air, and by sweating. Sweating in a sauna or steam bath is particularly effective.

You will also want to consider doing a complete bowel detoxification program. Sandy did it all. With four teenage sons to raise, she was scared, but ready to do whatever it took!

SANDY'S STORY AS TOLD BY RON LOWRIE
"SANDY'S DOWN TIMES BEGAN TO STRETCH OUT"

"It began with noticeable episodes of memory loss and numbness on her left side. Symptoms would change location from time to time, but numbness, tingling, and muscle weakness were becoming more and more noticeable. Then came an ever so slight dragging of her left leg. When it spread to the right side of her body, Sandy knew she needed help. Sandy certainly did not look like a person who had been given a diagnosis of probable MS (multiple sclerosis). All other possibilities had now been ruled out after two years of progressive symptoms and countless tests.

As a child, Sandy had played on soccer fields all over Washington state. One, very near an industrial cement plant in Tacoma belched toxic debris into the atmosphere daily. It was on the adjacent grounds that she had gained soccer skills good enough to receive a full-ride college scholarship and to participate in the U.S. Olympic Festival, earning gold medals while playing with winning teams throughout the 1980s.

I knew from my studies that people with heavy metal poisoning exhibited some symptoms similar to hers. I also knew she had a mouthful of silver (mercury) fillings and that completing a total body detoxification program (herbs, fiber, colonics, raw foods, juicing, and all the rest) could benefit her. And I was pretty sure that she would benefit from seeing a health-conscious dentist who knew about the problems of mercury. See the Appendix for more information on mercury.

I showed Sandy numerous environmental and dental reference books that contained scientific information about the issues of mercury toxicity. Then I told her about the renowned Seattle dentist who understood these issues. Months went by.

When Sandy became bedridden again, her husband Dan went to the internet in frustration. He wanted to see if there might be a nutritional approach to MS. Thinking about the mercury in her teeth, he found a Seattle dentist, Dr. Paul Genung (www.toothwisdom.net), who practiced health-conscious dentistry. Call it providence—it was the same dentist I'd told him about months prior.

Sandy worked hard at her recovery. Mercury fillings removal, medically supervised colonics, examinations and lab tests, lymphatic cleansings to help keep the toxins moving out of her body, and specific supplements helped purge the heavy metals (oral chelation). She also started eating a nutrient-dense, natural diet.

Sandy's times between down times began to stretch out. Over a few months, she was up more and more, looking and feeling healthier, and generally on the road to a full recovery. She knew she had had a breakthrough when she was able to run five miles with a friend. Her health and vitality were returning! Two years later, Sandy remains healthy and free of symptoms.

Toxicity from environmental pollutants almost destroyed this normally vibrant, energetic, and athletic woman. Learning about the toxic hazards of the twenty-first century, then deciding to do something about it, may well have saved her life!"

——

We'll begin with understanding how important internal cleanliness is and how bowel toxicity can cause ill health.

A TOXIC BOWEL MAY BE AT THE ROOT OF ILL HEALTH

Many of us have been taught by conventional medicine that elimination of food residue every three days is normal. We assume that our intestines are like a stainless-steel holding tank for toxic waste.

One of the most common signs of a toxic colon is chronic constipation. Constipation is a condition where the fecal matter is so tightly packed together that bowel movements are infrequent and incomplete. A toxic colon also becomes a breeding ground for parasites and worms.

Most experts in the field of natural health believe that elimination should occur at least once daily and possibly more frequently. Many say that having a bowel movement after every meal is ideal.

Dr. Bernard Jensen, D.C., PhD, author of numerous health books, was a leader in the field of detoxification for good health. According to Dr. Jensen:

> In the 50 years I've spent helping people to overcome illness, disability, and disease, it has become crystal clear that poor bowel management lies at the root of most people's health problems. In treating over 300,000 patients, the bowel invariably has to be cared for first before any effective healing can take place.[207]

Harvey W. Kellogg, M.D., states:

> "Of the 22,000 operations I performed personally, I've never found a single normal colon, and of the 100,000 performed under my jurisdiction, not over six percent were normal." [208]

The late Norman Walker, D.Sc., PhD, one of the twentieth century's most recognized colon experts, explains that the elimination of undigested food and other waste products is as important as the proper digestion and assimilation of food. It is his opinion that the failure to effectively eliminate waste products from the body causes so much fermentation and putrefaction in the colon that the neglected accumulation of such waste can, and frequently does, result in all kinds of diseases.

Ann Louise Gittleman, health expert, writes:

> In my opinion, we are not going to change the catastrophic situation where every second person is chronically ill until we place as much emphasis on internal cleansing as we do on external hygiene, such as brushing our teeth or washing our hands. If you are middle-aged, you've taken about 15,000 showers in your lifetime, and you've brushed your teeth close to 30,000 times. Still, you won't stop doing that just because you've done it so many times. Here's an interesting question: If you have to cleanse your teeth and body everyday, doesn't it makes sense to cleanse the inside of your body at least periodically?[209]

Robert O. Young, ND, says,

> Regular consumption by most North Americans of coffee and alcoholic beverages, and of low-nutrient, low-bulk, processed ingestibles is a doomsday habit. Over time, it transforms a healthy large intestine into a death-dealing pipe containing layers of encrusted fecal/mucoid material and debris—thereby promoting the over-growth of yeast and fungus and other morbid microforms. Vegetables are not mucoid-forming, which is just one more reason to make them the major portion of your diet.[210]

UNINVITED HOUSEGUESTS

We humans can actually play host to more than a hundred different types of parasites, ranging in size from microscopic to tapeworms that are several feet long. Contrary to what most people would think, parasites are not restricted to the colon alone, nor are they a problem that is confined to third-world countries. They can be found in any other part of the body—in the lungs, the liver, in the muscles and joints, in the esophagus, the brain, the blood, the skin, and even the eyes.

The occurrence of parasitic infestation in North America is on the rise due to globalization. In a recent parasite study involving 2,896 patients at the Parasitology Center in Tempe, Arizona, Dr. Omar Amin found one third of the patients tested positive for parasites involving 18 different species. [211]

CONDITIONS RELATED TO A TOXIC COLON

Most of the experts that I have quoted above agree that many unanswered health questions could be directly related to a toxic colon. There are numerous conditions that can be related in some way. Here is a partial list:

Acid reflux
Bloating
Candida
Constipation
Diverticulosis
Gas
Headache
Irritable bowel syndrome
Parasites
Protruding stomach
Stomach pain
Weight gain

Maybe you have struggled with these or similar problems, and tried everything to get better—laxatives, over-the-counter or prescription drugs, or even natural supplements. If you are still suffering, perhaps the root of the problem was never eliminated!

From Sandy's problem with mercury toxicity (above) to issues related directly to the bowel, a total body detoxification program is generally beneficial. There are numerous general cleanse kits that are easy to use and have some degree of effectiveness. Such a kit will include herbs that promote detoxification of the digestive system organs and support all elimination organs and systems: the bowels, the kidneys, lungs, skin, liver, blood, and lymphatic system.

Such cleansing kits are available at *www.gethealthyamerica.biz.*

ACTION PLAN FOR COLON HEALTH
GENERAL RECOMMENDATIONS

- Colonics, also called colon irrigation and colon hydrotherapy, is a method of washing out the colon using warm, purified water to help eliminate stored fecal matter, gas, mucus, and toxic substances. Colonics are performed in a professional setting with a trained colon therapist.

- Detox baths are good; you will find many variations of soak baths in books and on the internet. Here is one that Ron Lowrie likes: one cup sea salt, one cup Epsom salts, one cup baking soda, 1 to 2 heaping tbsp. ground/powdered ginger.

- Saunas: Used by many cultures, saunas are a powerful method of eliminating environmental chemicals that are stored in fat cells. Pregnant women should always consult a doctor.

DIETARY TIPS

- Consume anti-parasitic foods including onions, carrot tops, radish roots, kelp, raw cabbage, ground almonds, blackberries, pumpkin, sauerkraut, fresh pineapple, fresh papaya, and figs.

- Divide your weight in half, and drink that many ounces of water every day (if you weigh 140 pounds, you would drink seventy ounces of water). Water is critical to the effectiveness of any colon-cleansing program and to overall health.

BENEFICIAL VITAMINS, MINERALS, AND HERBS

Probiotics are beneficial bacteria normally found in the digestive tract. They are important for proper digestion and prevention of yeast overgrowth. A very high quality probiotic is available at *www.gethealtyamerica.biz.*

Fiber— As a supplement, it helps prevent colon problems by keeping food moving rapidly through the intestines.

Parasite Cleansing:— There are many parasite-cleansing formulas available in natural food stores. They contain various herbs and other nutrients that have parasite-killing properties. The herbs may include dandelion, milk thistle, mullein, burdock, corn silk, wormwood, garlic, cascara sagrada, flaxseed, rhubarb, black walnut hulls, Pau D'Arco, yellow dock, pumpkin seed, grapefruit extract, senna, fenugreek, cloves, slippery elm, or any combination of these. Carefully follow the directions on the product you choose to get maximum benefit.

Diatomaceous Earth— Composed of the fossilized shells of tiny water organisms called diatoms. They are found in many ancient seabeds throughout the world. Diatomaceous Earth acts like ground glass on the parasites and kills them without poisons or any upset to your system while doing no harm to humans. Diatomaceous earth is also a good mineral supplement. It is often used as a maintenance food to keep you parasite-free. It mixes with water or juice and is tasteless. This is available at *www.gethealthyamerica.biz.*

GET HEALTHY, AMERICA!

DIGESTIVE TRACT JUICE

Detox Delight
   1 small beet
   ½ lemon with or without peel
   ½ garlic clove
   1 handful of dandelion greens
   1 handful cilantro
   1 handful parsley

- Run ingredients through a juicer and drink immediately.

39 New Ideas—New Steps— New Habits

If a turn-of-the-century American could be propelled into a modern supermarket, he would be staggered by the vast quantity of available products—thousands instead of the 100 or so carried in his general store. Dazzled by the shiny, transparent plastics and colorful metallic packages, he might well think that he'd entered the Garden of Eden. Unfortunately, our abundance has led to a whole host of degenerative diseases, conclusively linked to nicely packaged but nutrient-deficient food.

Thanks to flashy, persuasive TV advertising, compounded by tight schedules and little time to shop, we mindlessly toss these foods into our carts. Week after week and year after year, we buy what we've always bought, healthy or not, and another week of eating and feeding begins.

You have probably heard the expression that "The definition of insanity is doing the same things over and over again and expecting different results!" If you have read this far in the book, maybe you are ready for a new way of doings things.

In this section, you will learn how to pick the healthiest foods possible from the thousands of choices available. If you are pursuing a path of renewed health, energy, and vigor, then walk away from the flashy abundance, and toward whole, natural foods. It's all about new ideas, new steps, and new habits.

Jim was in to the Tahoma Clinic to see Dr. Wright because he simply didn't feel good. After a complete history and physical, he was sent to the allergy department to be tested for food and chemical sensitivities. The day after his appointment, food allergy list in hand, he was in my office. Jim was ready to start a new journey, one of good health—albeit slowly—but as the expression goes, "How do you eat an elephant? One bite at a time."

JIM'S STORY

"LONG-HAUL TRUCKING AND EATING GOOD JUST DON'T MIX"

Jim was a long-haul trucker. His schedule had him on the road most of the time, and he consumed almost all of his meals at truck stops. The little time he was at home, he opted for pizza delivery, Chinese take out, or fast food. Jim came into the clinic with fatigue, severe headaches, and suspicion of allergies, since he noticed that he would get sleepy and headachy after eating.

Dr. Wright ordered allergy testing, specific lab tests, and nutritional IV therapy along with several supplements. After his appointment and visit to the allergy department, Jim was in to see me for help with his diet. Sure enough, his allergy screening showed that he was reactive to many foods, including what I call the big five—wheat, milk, corn, soy, and eggs.

"I'm happy and discouraged all at once," Jim said. "I'm glad to know that my problems weren't strictly mental. But it is discouraging to think of what foods I can't eat."

I assured Jim that we could plan a four-day-rotation diet that would help him get better (see allergy section).

He paused. "How am I going to do that? Do you know that I am a long-haul truck driver?"

"It won't be the easiest task you've ever undertaken," I said. "But it is not easy to feel bad all the time, either."

I started to explain how a rotation diet works and marked what foods he shouldn't eat at all for now and what foods he could eat on a rotation basis. I explained that foods that are only moderately reactive could usually be tolerated every four days as it takes about that long for the body to totally clear a food.

Jim looked me straight in the eye and let me know what he was thinking. "Forget it! It won't work, and I'll never do that. Impossible!"

"Well, Jim, then how can I help you?" I asked. "Would you like to just talk a little about a healthier diet?"

"Sure. I'll listen, but remember what I said: trucking and healthy diet—next to impossible."

I understood Jim's frustration and wanted to help him, but I could see he wasn't going to cooperate with what I requested. Frankly, it's not that easy to follow a rotation diet, even when you are home all the time and have a mate who is helping prepare food.

I put my pen down and looked at him. "Jim, what do you think you could do? Could you stop eating wheat? It's in breads, pastas, pies, cakes, cookies, and the like."

"I don't know how I could do that. Everything I eat at a truck stop is what you just said."

"Could you stop dairy products? Milk, yogurt, ice cream, and the like?"

"That sounds easier, but I can't guarantee it. What if something I eat has milk in it, and I don't even know it?"

Jim was being really nice during the conversation and very honest. But I could see he was not a willing participant in any allergy diet plan.

"Well, Jim, looking at what you told me you eat on an average day, I think maybe we could start with some minor diet changes. Do you eat fruit and vegetables?'

"The canned corn and peas at truck stops and sometimes a salad. I hardly ever eat fruit."

"Could you eat an apple a day?" I asked.

"That I could do! An apple a day!"

Finally, I got a commitment out of Jim. It was a small step, and it really wasn't dealing with his food allergies at all. But it was a step in the right direction. I never saw Jim after that, and I have often wondered how he was doing. I've always taught that the journey of a thousand miles begins with one-step.

——

Hopefully, that apple a day was the first step for Jim in beginning a healthier diet that could improve his quality of life and longevity. Maybe someday he'll tackle the allergies and rotation diet.

40 A New Way to Shop

Shop the periphery of the grocery store first, where you will find a bigger selection of unprocessed foods. I call them one ingredient foods—chicken breasts, potatoes, apples, broccoli, almonds, cheese, eggs, etc.

You will want to shop the inside aisles prudently because therein are the processed foods: commercial pastries, TV dinners, processed cheeses, potato chips, crackers, cookies, ice-cream, toaster pop-ups, artificial fruit drinks, soft drinks, and sugary cereals.

Keep in mind that when you buy processed foods, it is hard to tell what all you are eating, but almost for sure, you will be eating artificial colors, flavors, and preservatives.

BREAD AISLE—BUY 100% WHOLE GRAIN BREADS

If it says wheat bread, it is probably white flour with color added. When a loaf of bread costs $1.00 or less—even three for a dollar—it is probably not made from whole grains. Buy breads that say 100% whole-grain. If you are allergic to wheat, buy sprouted grain bread, rye bread, or spelt bread. You can find whole-grain substitutes for almost anything—pies, cakes, cookies, crackers, pasta products, and baked goods. Check out your local health food store.

BULK FOOD BINS—BUY NUTS, SEEDS, & WHOLE GRAINS

Here you will find a good selection of whole foods: nuts, seeds, beans, brown rice, oatmeal, whole-wheat pasta, trail mix, etc. Learn to cook beans and to sprout seeds. Buy a cookbook if you don't know how to sprout seeds or how to cook beans. These are very healthy and inexpensive foods. For sprouters, see *www.gethealthyamerica.biz*

THE CANNED GOODS AISLE— USE MINIMALLY

There are some canned goods that you will probably want to stock: tomato products, mushrooms, whole beans, and healthy soups. Don't buy canned vegetables, cheap soups, or highly sugared fruit. Buy your fruits and vegetables in the fresh produce section.

CEREAL AISLE—BUY NATURAL, WHOLE-GRAIN CEREALS & BREAKFAST FOODS

Buy no and low sugared cereals made from whole-grains. Health food stores carry an excellent selection, and they are generally cheaper because they are not highly advertised. Learn to make your own granola and make it in a large batch so it will last a while. Seal tightly and store in refrigerator.

Look below at the ingredients in two top-selling granola bars. Of the two choices, which do you think is the healthiest?

Popular Grocery Store Granola Bar: filling (high fructose corn syrup, corn syrup, mixed berry [strawberry, blueberry, raspberry] puree concentrates, apple puree concentrate, glycerin, sugar, natural flavor, modified corn starch, sodium alginate, sodium citrate, citric acid, malic acid, modified cellulose, dicalcium phosphate, red no. 40, blue No. 1), enriched flour (wheat flour, niacinamide, reduced iron, thiamin mononitrate [vitamin B1], riboflavin [vitamin B2], folic acid), whole grain oats, sugar, sunflower oil, high-fructose corn syrup, contains two percent or less of honey, calcium carbonate, dextrose, nonfat dry milk, wheat bran, salt, cellulose, potassium bicarbonate (leavening), natural and artificial flavor, mono and diglycerides, propylene glycol esters of fatty acids, soy lecithin, wheat gluten, cornstarch, vitamin A palmitate, carrageenan, niacinamide, sodium stearyl lactylate, guar gum, zinc oxide, reduced iron, pyridoxine hydrochloride (vitamin B6), thiamin hydrochloride (vitamin B1), riboflavin (vitamin B2), folic acid.

Popular Granola from a Natural food Store: oats, coconut, honey, sunflower seeds, canola oil, ground flax, wheat bran, wheat germ, sesame seeds, pure vanilla extract, sea salt.

CONDIMENT AISLE

Many of the products in this aisle are fairly healthy—mustard, pickles, olives, peppers, etc. However, catsup, mayonnaise, and salad dressings have sugar and preservatives. Check out the health food store for healthier choices.

DAIRY AISLE

If you use dairy milk, look for a brand that is organic and hormone-free. Try dairy alternatives like almond, rice, and soy milk or even oat milk. You can readily find organic or soy yogurts that are sweetened with natural sweeteners.

FROZEN FOODS AISLE—BUY VEGETABLES, FRUITS & UNSWEETENED JUICES

Buy juices that say 100% pure juice. Don't buy varieties that contain sugar. Stock up on unsweetened frozen fruits of all sorts for smoothies or dessert sauces. Frozen fruits and vegetables are picked at the height of the season and flash frozen so they are a good second choice. They are far superior to canned fruits and vegetables and the next best choice after fresh.

MEAT & FISH AISLE—BUY ORGANIC, LEAN CUTS

If you eat meat, try eating less, making it more of a condiment than the main course. Use it sparingly in stir-fry dishes that have plenty of vegetables. Try to find organic sources. Look for local farms in your area. Buy wild salmon rather than farmed-raised. It is notably higher in nutrients. I do not recommend eating pork because of health issues surrounding it.

OIL & SHORTENING AISLE—DON'T BUY!

Don't buy any products listing partially hydrogenated oil as an ingredient, regardless of the type of oil, and don't use vegetable shortenings or similar hardened fats. By following these rules, you will be avoiding transfats.

Don't buy margarine, regardless of health claims made by the manufacturer. Buy olive oil, ghee (clarified butter), pure butter, and other cold-pressed oils from a natural food store. To stretch butter, try making "better butter," which remains spreadable even after refrigeration: mix ½ butter and ½ olive or flax oil. Place in a container and store in the refrigerator.

PACKAGED FOOD AISLE— CAKES & BAKERY GOODS

These are all made with white flour and sugar. If you bake from scratch, buy a cookbook that tells you how to use whole-wheat flour and honey. The natural food section of your store will carry bakery goods—packaged or ready made—with natural ingredients.

PRODUCE AISLE—BUY PLENTY— & ORGANIC, WHEN POSSIBLE

Fill your cart with fruits and vegetables. Buy a juicer, and begin to make a juice a day, using lots of dark, leafy-green vegetables: collards, Romaine, kale, Swiss chard, parsley, cilantro, etc. Get rid of the nutrient-deficient iceberg lettuce and use these healthy greens instead. Introduce new fruits and vegetables into the family diet in addition to the ones you normally buy: mango, persimmons, pomegranate, and ugly fruit.

EAT MORE ALKALINE & LESS ACID FOODS

The Standard American Diet—high in meat, sugar, alcohol, coffee, fish, milk, noodles, pasta, shellfish, and eggs—is highly acid-forming, which means it pushes the body chemistry toward the acid side. In general, disease is associated with an over-acid body, and many naturally-oriented healthcare practitioners feel that a diet that contains more alkaline-forming than acid-forming foods promotes health and helps ward off diseases. A good rule is to make the diet 80% alkaline-forming foods and only 20% acid-forming foods. Don't go overboard; you need some acid foods in the diet for balance.

What this means in real life choices is that you should eat less meat, dairy, fish, and poultry (all of which leave an acid ash in the body once they're metabolized) and more fruits and vegetables (which generally leave an alkaline ash). As a rule of thumb, fill only ¼ of your plate with acid-forming foods and ¾ of it with alkaline-forming foods.

Acid-Forming Foods: Alcohol, asparagus, beans, Brussels sprouts, buckwheat, catsup, chickpeas, cocoa, coffee, cornstarch, cranberries, eggs, fish, flour, legumes, lentils, meat, milk, mustard, noodles, oatmeal, olives, pasta, pepper, plums, poultry, prunes, shellfish, soft drinks, sugar, tea, and vinegar.

Alkaline-Forming Foods: Avocados, corn, dates, fresh coconut, fresh fruits (most), honey, horseradish, maple syrup, molasses, mushrooms, onions, raisins, soy products, sprouts, umeboshi plums, and watercress.

4️⃣1️⃣ Developing Healthy Habits

I heard this simple little story somewhere along the way and think it is very appropriate here. It is called, A Five Chapter Story.

Chapter One: I was walking down the road. There was a big hole in the sidewalk. I didn't see it. I fell in. It wasn't my fault. No one helped me get out. I finally got out on my own. It took me a long time.

Chapter Two: I was walking down the same road. There was a big hole in the sidewalk. I saw it. I fell in anyway. It wasn't my fault. I got out quickly.

Chapter Three: I was walking down the road. I saw the big hole in the sidewalk. I tried to avoid it but fell in. It was my fault. I got out quickly.

Chapter Four: I was walking down the road. I walked around the big hole.

Chapter Five: I took another road.

Perhaps you have reached a point in your life where you are ready to take another road—maybe a road of renewed health. I've found in life that sometimes the best direction to go is 180 degrees from the direction I was heading. Maybe you have already incorporated many of the suggestions in this book. Hopefully, you will find something on this list that will be of further benefit.

TAKE DEEP BREATHS EVERYDAY

Notice how shallow your normal daily breathing is. Get in the habit of taking deep breathes everyday. Practice by placing your hands on your stomach and inhaling slowly and deeply through your nose. You should feel the air going deep into your stomach. Exhale, then begin the inhale-exhale cycle again. Repeat the breaths several times daily.

AVOID OR NEUTRALIZE ELECTRONIC GADGETS

A growing body of evidence has shown that electromagnetic radiation emitted from cell phones, cordless phones, iPods, PDA's, computers, Bluetooth, and microwaves can have devastating effects on health and may increase risks for disease over time. Called *electropollution,* many experts think it is one of the greatest health risks of the twenty-first century.

Research has associated use of these devises with increased risks of brain cancer, headaches, nausea, and muscle pain. There are devices available that attach directly to these objects and greatly reduce exposure to this electromagnetic toxin. You can get more information at *www.gethealthyamerica.biz.*

EXERCISE HABITUALLY

This topic has been worked to death so I won't expound, other than to say you should be doing something that gets you moving.

FORGIVENESS

A dear friend gave me a wall plaque many years ago that read, "Forgiveness is the fragrance that the flower leaves on the heel of the boot that crushes it." Over the years, I've thought about that plaque and have come to realize that being mad at someone or having unforgiveness doesn't hurt that person—it just hurts me. I've also learned the need to forgive, even if the other person was wrong. This doesn't make the wrong right, it simply frees you up from the negative emotion. As the saying goes, "Let go, and let God."

"Forbearing one another, and forgiving one another, if any man have a quarrel against any: even as Christ forgave you, so also do ye." Colossians 3:13 (KJV)

LAUGH FOR HEALTH

In his book *Anatomy of an Illness,* Norman Cousins describes how watching Marx Brother's movies helped him recover from a life-threatening disease. He wondered if it was possible that love, hope, faith, and laughter could be of any value. He said he enjoyed a hearty belly laugh several times a day and that the laugher gave him relief from pain.

Laughter seems to positively affect heart health, as a University of Maryland Medical Center study recently showed. People with heart disease were 40% less likely to laugh compared to people without heart disease. Researchers aren't sure why this occurs, but theorize it has to do with laughter's ability to lessen the effects of mental stress.[212]

"Then was our mouth filled with laughter, and our tongue with singing:" Psalms 126:2a,b (KJV)

POSITIVE ATTITUDE

Even hard science says that not only can having a positive attitude improve our mental health but that it can also keep us physically fit. Recent studies done by the University of Texas found that people with an upbeat view of life were less likely than pessimists to show signs of frailty. They also delayed the aging process! Over a seven-year period, researchers assessed over 1,500 older people for frailty (weight loss, exhaustion, walking speed, and grip strength). They found that those people who had a positive attitude towards life were significantly less likely to show these signs of frailty.

"Whatsoever things are true, whatsoever things are honest, whatsoever things are just, whatsoever things are pure, whatsoever things are lovely, whatsoever things are of good report; if there be any virtue, and if there be any praise, think on these things." Philippians 4:8 (KJV)

EAT LIGHTLY BEFORE RETIRING

It has been said that you should eat like a king for breakfast, a queen for lunch, and a pauper for dinner. Since digestion slows down when you sleep, it's a good idea not go to bed with a heavy meal on your stomach. In several scientific studies, it was recently reported that people who eat 25% less than the average person of their height are more likely to live to be 100!

EAT MORE RAW FOODS

Adding more raw foods to your diet is a great starting place to move toward better health. Eat at least 50% of your diet as raw fruits, vegetables, nuts, and seeds. You will never find a study that says people became healthier by eating candy, pastry, TV dinners, or by guzzling soft drinks. Raw foods are high in nutrition and natural enzymes that make digestion easier.

"I have given you every herb bearing seed, which is upon the face of all the earth, and every tree, in the which is the fruit of a tree yielding seed; to you it shall be for meat." Genesis 1:29 (KJV)

REST

God commands rest—a time to recover emotionally, physically, and spiritually. Take one day in seven and enjoy the national parks, the ocean, or just a backyard BBQ. Or do something fun with the family.

"And God blessed the seventh day, and sanctified it: because that in it he had rested from all his work which God created and made."

Genesis 2:3 (KJV)

"Remember the sabbath day, to keep it holy. Six days shalt thou labour, and do all thy work: But the seventh day is the Sabbath of the LORD thy God: in it thou shalt not do any work, thou, nor thy son, nor thy daughter, thy manservant, nor thy maidservant, nor thy cattle, nor thy stranger that is within thy gates."

Exodus 20:8–10 (KJV)

SLEEP

Scientists have found that only when it's really dark can your body produce the hormone called melatonin. *Melatonin* (the hormone that regulates the sleep-wake cycle) fights diseases, including breast and prostate cancer.

Researchers in this field say that lack of sleep or being subjected to light at night instead of complete darkness increases health risks. Even a little light around your bed at night can cause melatonin production to switch off. The two to three hours before midnight provide the greatest window of opportunity for the repair and healing of the body.

"I will both lay me down in peace, and sleep: for thou, LORD only makest me dwell in safety." Psalms 4:8 (KJV)

"...for so he giveth his beloved sleep." Psalms 127:2d (KJV)

WATER

To understand the importance of drinking water, you will want to read, *Your Body's Many Cries for Water* by F. Batmanghelidj, MD. He writes that your body must have adequate amounts of water in order to function properly. The body is 75% water, which means that a constant supply is imperative for maintaining optimum health. Chronic dehydration has been shown to be directly related to nearly all human disease.[213]

Whatever water you drink, it is critical that you drink enough and that it is pure. See *www.gethealthyamerica.biz* to learn about an innovative countertop, alkalizing water system, and pocket sized wands that are water enhancing and restructuring.

"Whether therefore ye eat, or drink, or whatsoever ye do, do all to the glory of God. 1 Corinthians 10:31 (KJV)

While some people make changes quickly, Katrina began her journey slowly but steadily.

KATRINA'S STORY—

MY PATH TO HEALTH (DAUGHTER OF RON LOWRIE)

"I LOVE TO HELP OTHERS ON THEIR PATH TO HEALTH"

"I was raised on a pretty traditional American diet. Mom always made healthy meals by normal standards—noodles, casseroles, meat, potatoes, and the like. On holidays, her culinary skills shined from her years of working in the banquet industry. Family affairs were lavish with the best the season had to offer. I remember when my dad began to look at healthier options, but at the time, none of us were particularly interested.

My parents divorced when I was twelve, and it was very painful for me. I was an adult before I realized how much unforgiveness and resentment I had from the divorce. Because of this, I would hear nothing of my Dad's suggestions to "follow a healthier lifestyle."

Then came marriage, pregnancy, and a whole new perspective on life. I wanted my best, and God's best, for my unborn child, and I knew that it would mean some spiritual, as well as dietary changes.

My willing husband and I started on our new path to health, slowly at first, just a little at a time—baby steps in preparation for the baby. But we were determined.

I began reading and searching the internet. I learned that cows were injected with genetically engineered hormones that caused them to give up to 15% more milk, and that little girls today are reaching puberty far earlier very possibly because of these hormones. I was concerned for my unborn child, so switching to non-dairy cheese and milk alternatives was easy. Besides, I never felt very good from dairy products, and I like the rice, almond, and soy alternatives better anyway.

Then I learned how sugar depresses the immune system and how it can lead to diabetes and heart problems, and that the average American ate two to three pounds of it a week. I found numerous sugar-free treats at my local natural food stores. Sweetened with pure fruit juice, honey, or the herb stevia, they were far healthier and could be eaten in moderation. Again, I thought how these were better choices for my child and husband.

Over time, we weaned ourselves off sugar, most processed foods, dairy products, and the like. About a year into our diet change adventure, I had a craving for some pizza. Of course I indulged myself. That pizza knotted up my stomach so badly, I lay on the couch for two days in a lot of discomfort. I'd learned my lesson.

Because I am outgoing by nature and passionate about what I've learned, I frequently share ideas with friends. They often ask me, "How can I get started?" I tell them to start by eliminating one unhealthy food that they can live without—say soft drinks, or the daily candy bar, or maybe the latte they have every morning (which, by the way, has upwards of 500 calories in the creamy varieties).

I ask them if they know that red dye #40 has been shown to cause behavior problems in children and that it is in many baked goods, candies, and soft drinks they give their children. Then I suggest they read the ingredients listed on the label of the TV dinners they frequently eat.

People complain that it's too expensive to eat healthy. I respond by informing them that it is more expensive to eat the traditional way we call the Standard American Diet (SAD). A big bag of potato chips costs up to $4.00. I call it a bag of "unfood." For the same $4.00, they could buy a big bag of apples. Spread apple slices with almond butter and sprinkle with coconut, and you have a very healthy snack that is good for you.

Nuts are a good snack (unsalted and un-oiled) and you can buy a whole bag for about the price of a latte or double-dip ice cream cone. And think how long that bag will last compared to the coffee and cone, not to mention the digestive benefits to chewing rather than just gulping food.

I teach people to shop the outside aisles. This is where you will find foods that are the least processed—fresh fruits and vegetables, seafood, meat, and bins of bulk foods like nuts, grains, and healthier snacks. Generally, the center aisles are full of highly processed, prepared, and packaged foods that may be convenient, but are packed with unhealthy ingredients. Just read the labels.

I ask them to notice the eye-level positioning of the brand name cereals and goodies their children love. Hmmm? Could the manufacturers and advertisers be up to something?

God has blessed me with two beautiful children that I learned early to feed well. They rarely get sick, and the few times they have been ill, they've recovered quickly. Seasonally, I watch as my friends give their children antibiotics for colds and ear infections—several times a year. I always suggest that they change their family's diet.

Recently, a friend who was watching my children made them a peanut butter and jelly sandwich on white bread. They had never tasted white bread, and they didn't like it one bit! They said it was too gooey, so my friend had to give them apples instead.

We all deserve to have healthy, happy children, and a happy spouse as well. I believe our lifestyle changes have helped us move toward achieving this milestone as a family. I do not say this to brag, rather to perhaps help someone else realize that they too can start on their own health journey, give their children strong, healthy bodies, and hope for a bright future. In the classes I teach, we cover the simplicity of full circle health—striving for balance between body, mind, and spirit."

Remember that familiar saying, "A journey of a thousand miles begins with the first step." Our American culture seems confused and appears out of control regarding what constitutes good health. We just might want to think about returning to a simpler life. Maybe an apple a day will indeed keep the doctor away."

—

Note: Katrina Lowrie-Fernandez is the Florida representative for Get Healthy, America! She is available to teach her seminar, "Full Circle Health," to local home groups and women's church associations. Contact *www.gethealthyamerica.biz* for more information.

4 2 The Eat Clean Move More Lifestyle

I was a ballet dancer from the time I was four years old until I was twenty and even auditioned for American Ballet Theatre in New York City. My dancing career, which led up to that professional audition, was riddled with weight problems. Mostly, it was just an extra five pounds, but dressed in a tutu as the Sugar Plum Fairy, those extra pounds really made a difference.

So I began the whole diet routine at the age of twelve. I tried it all—the cottage cheese diet, the grapefruit diet, the Atkins diet, the Dr. Stillman diet (mostly meat and lots of water), the banana diet (I actually gained five pounds on this one), and simply going without any food. I also experimented with the first weight-loss shake Metracal (anyone old enough to remember this?) and Ayds, the individually wrapped caramel candy that was supposed to expand in your stomach when you drank a hot cup of tea.

When I decided to become a flight attendant rather than dance, at age twenty-one, the maximum weight allowed for my height of 5'5" was 129 pounds. Weight check took place at the beginning of each month, and if you were even ¼ a pound over, you were grounded. Then you were sent immediately to the company doctor to see "what your problem was." The Continental Airlines physician, Dr. Rosenfeld in Seattle, told me I had mild obesity (I weighed 131 pounds), then handed me a 1000-calorie-a-day diet plan. I was stunned and said, "Dr. Rosenfeld, mild obesity?" "It's just a medical term," he said. I've never forgotten it!

Like me, I am sure that many of the baby boomers feel like they've done it all with dieting and are through with the whole routine. But whether you are a baby boomer or not, if your goal is good health and reasonable weight, then following the basic principles in this book will be to your benefit. I summarize it simply and concisely by saying, "Eat clean, move more."

Eating clean means making the majority of your diet selections from whole, unprocessed foods. I call them one-ingredient foods. One-ingredient foods are things like an apple, a salmon steak, a handful of almonds, an egg, or broccoli. They are the kinds of foods you have read about in this book.

Move more means just that: Get up and start moving! I recommend buying a pedometer (see index) so you can track your daily steps. You will most likely find that if you follow a normal daily routine, you will never reach the 10,000 steps recommended by health experts. To reach that goal, you will need to take a walk, go to the gym, or do some other form of exercise.

Whether you are just starting on a path to good health or have been on your journey for a long time, eat clean and move more! Listed below are "eating clean" foods specific to different body systems.

FOODS FOR A HEALTHY HEART & CIRCULATORY SYSTEM

Cold-water fish (salmon—wild is far superior), garlic, olive oil, hawthorn berry tea, raw nuts, blackstrap molasses, citrus fruits (eat as much of the white lining as you can for bioflavonoids), apples, dark leafy greens, and cayenne pepper.

FOODS FOR A GOOD BRAIN & SHARP MIND

Brazil nuts, blueberries, salmon, pears, apples, broccoli, spinach, lecithin, eggs, soybeans, pumpkin seeds, dark leafy greens, nuts, cheese, and lean meat.

FOODS FOR HEALTHY, STRONG BONES

Cold-water fish, horsetail tea, pineapple, apples, broccoli, soybeans, kelp, cherries, almonds, raisins, dates, beans, and dark leafy green vegetables.

FOODS FOR ANTI-AGING & NATURAL BEAUTY

Yogurt, kelp, pistachios, lecithin, oats, coconut, olive oil, beans, guava, dark leafy greens, chives, berries, persimmons, salmon, wheat germ, sesame seeds, carrots, eggs, spinach, peas, and brown rice.

FOODS FOR HEALTHY GLANDS & ORGANS

Dark leafy green vegetables, cherries, raw nuts, mushrooms, beets, lemons, high-fiber foods, raw foods, raw honey, apple cider vinegar, and walnuts.

FOODS FOR A HEALTHY DIGESTIVE TRACT

Raw foods, cloves, garlic, pumpkin seeds, lemons, beets, wheatgrass, black walnuts, papaya, watermelon, and onions.

PLANET EARTH POWER FOODS

Cold-water fish, lean meat, eggs, beans, garlic, olive oil, dark leafy greens, raw nuts, fruits with skins, root vegetables, and sprouted seeds.

As we come to the end of the book, remember that no one is perfect, and we all indulge from time to time. When that happens, don't give up! Just pick up where you left off, and continue with your new way of eating. Both immediate results and long-term health benefits will be your reward. It is all worth it!

I will leave with words of wisdom spoken, time and again, by our mentor and teacher, the late Elizabeth Baker. When people came out of the audience and asked her, "Elizabeth, what can I 'take' to be healthy?" Her answer was always the same. As she took their hands in hers, she would look them straight in the eyes and say, "My dear, you take the bad out of the diet!" So here's to your health, and congratulations on beginning your journey!

GLOSSARY

Abscisic Acid: an ingredient found in wheatgrass that is good for cancer prevention.

Acid Reflux: a condition in which acid flows back up from the stomach into the esophagus, causing pain.

Addiction: a compulsive activity and overwhelming involvement with a specific activity. May involve the use of almost any substance or a repetitive negative or destructive behavior.

Adrenal Glands: a pair of triangular-shaped organs that rest on top of the kidneys. Many of the stress hormones are produced here. Reduced adrenal function can result in weakness, lethargy, dizziness, memory problems and blood sugar disorders.

Adult Onset Diabetes: a type of diabetes in which patients are not dependent on injections of insulin. The disease usually begins after 40 years of age, but can occur at any age.

Aflatoxin: a cancer-causing mold found on foods like grains and nuts, particularly peanuts.

Agave Syrup: new in the marketplace, it comes from a cactus and has an excellent flavor. Used for sweeting foods. It is said to be low on the glycemic index.

Alkalinize: to make alkaline; 7.0 to 14.0 on the pH scale and opposite from acidic.

Allergen: any substance that causes manifestations of allergy.

Allergic Foods: foods that contain allergens and cause allergic reactions. Known culprits are corn, soy, wheat, dairy, peanuts, eggs, pollen, and nightshade foods like tomato, potato, eggplant, peppers, and tobacco.

Allopathic: a medical approach, which seeks to treat illness by producing a condition in the body that does not allow the disease to live or thrive. Allopathy is the commonly used medical method today.

Anaphylaxis/Anaphylactic Shock: sever reaction resulting from a substance to which an individual has become sensitized. For conservation and survival, the body begins to shut down and unless an antigen or medical treatment is administered immediately, it can result in death; e.g., snake bite, bee stings.

Angina: when the body is unable to pump blood as it should because of poor muscle contractions, the body receives signals from the heart in the form of pain.

Antacid: an agent that neutralizes stomach acid or acidity.

Apple Cider Vinegar: rich in multi-vitamin/minerals; overall tonic to boost immune system.

Ayurvedic: one of the oldest systems of holistic and preventive medicine from India that employs nutrition counselling, yoga, massage, herbal medicine, meditation and other modalities.

Bile: a digestive enzyme produced by the liver and stored in the gallbladder.

Bioflavonoid: a biologically active ingredient found in citrus and other fruits that provide health benefits against cancer and heart disease.

Biotin: related to the vitamin B family biotin keeps hair, skin and glands healthy.

Blood/Brain Barrier: a mechanism involving the capillaries and other cells of the brain that keep many substances from passing out of the blood vessels to be absorbed by the brain tissue.

Brewer's Yeast: the dried, pulverized cells of Saccharomyces cerevisiae, a type of fungus. It is a rich source of B-complex vitamins, protein (providing all essential amino acids), chromium, and minerals.

Bromelain: a natural enzyme and digestive aid found in pineapple.

Candida Albicans: a type of yeast that normally lives in the digestive tract and vagina and is kept in check by beneficial bacteria in the intestines.

Capillary Beds: the place where the blood of the arteries turns and goes into the veins.

Carcinogenic: producing cancer.

Cardiovascular Disease: a term that is used for heart attack, stroke, and other heart and blood vessel disorders.

Carotenoids: a class of compounds related to vitamin A that can act as precursors of vitamin A. Beta-carotene is the most widely known.

Celtic Salt: Celtic or Real Salt (the later = brand name) come from a hand crafted method of harvesting seawater off the Brittany coast, hence the name Celtic. It is naturally dried by the air and sun and retains all of the rich sea minerals of the ocean.

Choline: related to the vitamin B family, choline aids the liver and helps remove fat.

Cilia: hair like fibers present in the respiratory tract.

Cold Pressed Oil: a word applied to the least heat-treated process of extracting oil. The oil of seeds, grains or nuts is pressed out by large rollers. Considered a better choice than common grocery store-variety clear oils.

Colon: another name for the large intestine; also the lower bowel.

Curcumin: an ingredient in turmeric that stops inflammation and slows bone loss.

Degenerative Disease: a lifestyle disease as opposed to a communicable disease; the former a result of hereditary weaknesses, diet, and poor lifestyle.

Dental Caries: decay of the teeth.

Devitalized Foods: destruction or loss of vitamins and minerals.

Digestive Enzymes: chemicals produced in the stomach to help digest foods.

Diuretic: increasing or an agent that increases the secretion of urine.

Diverticulosis: big pockets pouching out in the wall of the large intestine.

Dopamine: a neurotransmitter produced in the brain and commonly associated with mood.

Edema: a local or generalized condition in which the body tissues contain an excessive amount of tissue fluid.

Eliminative Channels: skin, intestines, breath.

Enteric: coated with a material that permits transit through the stomach to the small intestine before the medication is released. Some probiotic supplements offer this delivery system so that stomach acids do not destroy the friendly bacteria.

Enzymes/Digestive Enzymes: chemicals responsible for the breakdown of foods.

Epigallocatechin gallate-EGCG: a powerful antioxidant found in green tea.

Expectorant: an agent that facilitates the removal of the secretions of the bronchopulmonary mucous membrane.

Fasting: temporarily abstaining from food. Usually only water is consumed for a period or hours or days.

Ferritin: (another name for iron).

Fermentation: the breakdown of carbohydrates by microorganisms. Fermented foods are one of the markers thought to contribute to longevity and optimal health among various cultures worldwide: e.g. natto, sauerkraut, keifer.

Fiber: components of food that are resistant to chemical digestion, including cellulose, hemicellulose, lignin, and pectin.

Flavonoids: (see bioflavonoid above).

Free Radical: atoms that cause damage to cells, impairing immune function, leading to infections and various degenerative diseases.

Full Spectrum Lighting: these lights emit a certain amount of ultra-violet as well as all colors in daylight from red to violet.

Galactomannan: active gel-like ingredient found in fenugreek.

Gluten: component of wheat, rye, oats, barley and related grains such as triticale and kamut; in susceptible people, the body responds to gluten as if it were an antigen, causing an allergic reaction.

Glycemic Index: a scale that ranks carbohydrate-rich foods by how much they raise blood glucose levels compared to glucose or white bread.

Herbicidal: chemical substances for killing unwanted plants.

Heidleberg Stomach Acid Test: a clinical procedure that measures stomach acid

Homeostasis: maintaining a stable condition in the body where all systems are in balance; the body's attempt to keep equilibrium between interrelated internal systems.

Hormones: a substance originating in an organ, gland, or part, which is conveyed through the blood to another part of the body, stimulating it by chemical action to increase activity or secretion of another hormone.

Hydrochloric Acid (HCl): the major digestive enzyme found in the stomach that breaks down proteins.

Hydrogenation: a chemical process where liquid fats have hydrogen atoms attached to make them solid; examples include margarine and shortening.

Hypericin: a medically active component found in St. John's Wort.

Immune System: that part of the body that reacts to substances that are foreign or are interpreted as being foreign. This involves lymphocytes, T-cells, B cells, phagocytes, suppressor cells or helper cells.

Inhibine: a bacteria-killing agent found in raw honey.

Insulin: a hormone made in the pancreas that controls the amount of glucose (sugar) in the blood and the rate at which glucose is absorbed into the cells.

Insulin Resistance: a condition in which the cells of the body become resistant to the effects of insulin. Higher levels of insulin are needed in order for insulin to have its effects.

Isothiocyanates: powerful phytochemicals that are anti-cancer.

Lecithin: mainly in eggs and soy; nerve cells/brain sheath composed of; needed by all body cells.

Lycopene: antioxidant; red pigment in tomatoes, pink grapefruit, watermelon; associated with lower risk of prostate cancer/cardio-vascular disease.

Manufactured Foods: foods that are radiated chemically injected, dyes added, fillers mixed in, and produced in mass quantities in commercial kitchens are manufactured foods; often referred to as "unfood."

Metabolic Syndrome: a constellation of metabolic disorders that all result from the primary disorder of insulin resistance.

Micronutrients: essential nutrients required only in small amounts.

Milligrams: one-thousandth of a gram.

Mucoid Plaque: accumulation of caked, layered encrusted fecal matter in the intestines.

Myelin Sheath: a multilayered, white, phospholipid-rich, segmented covering in the brain.

Naturopathic Physician: a discipline emphasizing prevention and treatment with the focus on self-healing, natural remedies, herbs, massage, midwifery acupuncture, etc.

Neurotransmitter: substance such as norepinephrine, acetycholine, and dopamine that is released in the brain.

Neural-Tube Defects: nerves or connected with the nervous system manifesting at birth.

Nightshade Plants: potato, tomato, eggplant, tobacco, peppers; chemical "solanine" may cause stiffness in arthritics.

Organic: means naturally occurring, with no chemicals used during growth.

Orthomolecular Psychiatry: means right molecule and the goal is to have a balanced metabolism by having the appropriate nutrition.

Pepsin: a digestive enzyme produced in the stomach.

Peristalsis: an automatic slow, wavelike motion that happens along the entire gastrointestinal tract that propels food along.

Pesticide: a manmade chemical used to control, repel, or destroy pests of any sort.

Phytochemicals: compounds present in plants that make the plants biologically active and determine color, flavor and its ability to resist disease.

Plaque: a patch on the skin or on a mucous surface. A yellow swollen area of the lining of an artery. In dentistry, a gummy mass of microorganisms that grows on the crowns and spreads along the roots of the teeth.

Polyphenol: a substance that is found in many plants and gives some flowers, fruits, and vegetables their color; they have antioxidant activity.

Postpartum: occurring after childbirth.

Poultice: a soft, moist mass of herbs or medicine that is spread on a cloth and applied externally to an inflamed area of the body.

Practitioner: one who has met the professional and legal requirements necessary to provide a health care service such as a physician, nurse, dentist or physicial therapist.

Probiotics: dietary supplements that contain beneficial bacteria such as acidophilus.

Ptyalin: an enzyme that begins the breakdown of carbohydrates in the mouth.

Purine: compounds in certain foods that create uric acid.

Quercetin: a bioflavonoid that reduces asthma symptoms, among other benefits.

Rancid/Rancidity: offensive, having a disagreeable smell or taste from partial decomposition, esp. of a fatty substance.

Raw Foods: any uncooked food, which is rich in enzymes, retains all original nutrients, digests easily and is powerful nutrition for healing.

Reactive Hypoglycemia: a medical term defined as "occurring 2–4 hours after a high carbohydrate meal (or oral glucose load)." It is thought to represent a consequence of excessive insulin release triggered by the carbohydrate meal but continuing past the digestion and disposal of the glucose derived from the meal.

Rebounding: a mini-trampoline about 30" to 40" inches in diameter that stimulates lymphatic movement and creates momentary weightlessness when airborne.

Reflexology: a science that deals with reflex points/meridians/locations in the feet, each of which is reflexively related to each organ in the body.

Roughage: found in plants, it is the fiber that cannot be digested but passes through the body, acting like an intestinal broom.

Rutin: an ingredient (buckwheat a rich source) which can strengthen the blood vessel walls.

Salivary Glands: produce saliva to moisten foods for swallowing and digestion.

Salves: selected herbs that are mixed into an oily or creamy base. They are formulated to penetrate the skin and are used externally.

Scurvy: a deficiency disease characterized by hemorrhagic manifestations and abnormal formation of bones and teeth.

Small Intestine: a long tube approximately one inch in diameter and 21 feet long. It begins at the stomach and ends where the large intestine begins. Most nutrient absorption happens here through the millions of finger-like projections called villi.

Sprouts: seeds that have been moistened and are growing; greatly increases nutrition; high in C.

Standard American Diet: called "SAD," it is a diet full of processed foods, chemically laced, dyed, hydrogenated, pasteurized, canned, frozen, nutrient stripped, etc.

Stevia: a natural herb sweetener, non-caloric and native to Paraguay.

Transfats: liquid fats that are made solid by the introduction of hydrogen. The purpose is to make a product that will spread.

Uric Acid: the end product of the metabolism of chemicals known as purines; associated with gout; when it crystallizes, it takes the shape of a needle and causes severe pain.

Vegan: someone who does not eat meat, fish, dairy products or eggs; often the indivdual will not wear anything that comes from an animal.

Vegetarian: someone who eats vegetables, seeds, tubers, fruit and grains and usually eggs and dairy products but not fish and meat.

Villi: fingerlike projections in the small intestine that aid absorption.

Wheatgrass: a rich nutritional beverage popularized by Dr. Ann Wigmore and containing a great variety of chlorophyll, vitamins, minerals and trace elements.

Zeaxanthin: in the family of carotenoids. Similar to other carotenoids, such as beta-carotene, lutein and alpha-carotene. Lycopenes cannot be produced by the body and therefore must be included in the diet.

BOOKS

ADD/ADHD
The Way They Learn by Cynthia Tobias, MED
Feed Your Kids Right by Leonard Smith, MD
Our Toxic World by Doris Rapp, MD
The Crazy Makers by Carol Simontacci, CCN

Addictions
Seven Weeks To Sobriety by Joan Mathews Larson, PhD
Under the Influence by James R. Milam, PhD

Allergy/Addiction
Single Food Stress Testing by Robert Bagley, PhD
Basics of Food Allergy by J.D. Breneman, MD
Tracking Down Hidden Food Allergies by William Crook, MD
Lick the Sugar Habit by Nancy Appleton, PhD
Is This Your Child? by Doris Rapp MD
The Allergy Self-Help Cookbook by Marjorie Hurt Jones
Kathy's Allergy-Ease Recipes by Kathy Parslow
See www.parentsofallergicchildren.org

Anti-Aging
Gary Null's Power Aging by Gary Null
Earl Mindell's Anti-Aging Bible by Earl Mindell

Blood/Body Chemistry
Blood Types, 4 Diets, Eat Right for Your Blood Type by

Peter J. D'Adamo, ND

Cancer

A Cancer Therapy: Results of Fifty Cases and the Cure of Advanced Cancer by Max Gerson
The Cure for All Cancers by Hulda Regehr Clark, PhD, ND
Surviving Cancer by Dee Simmons

Detoxification

Cleansing or Surgery by Paul Revere, Pastor (Embassy of Heaven)
Detoxify or Die by Sherry Rogers, MD
Tissue Cleansing Through Bowel Management by Bernard Jensen, D.C., PhD, Nutritionist

Digestion

Gut Solution by Brenda Watson, ND
Why Stomach Acid Is Good For You by Jonathan Wright, MD

Fasting

The Miracle of Fasting by Paul C. Bragg, ND, PhD

Fats

Fats that Heal, Fats that Kill: The Complete Guide to Fats, Oils, Cholesterol and Human Health by Edo Erasmus

General Health

Get Health Now! by Gary Null
Food–Your Miracle Medicine by Jean Carper
Folk Medicine by J.C. Jarvis
Eat Right. Live Longer by Neal Barnard MD
Prescription for Nutritional Healing by James and Phyllis Balch

The Terrain Is Everything by Susan Stockton
Your Body's Many Cries for Water by Feyedoon Batmanghelidj MD
Health and Light: The Effect of Natural and Artificial Light on Man and Other Living Things by John T. Ott
Heal Yourself With Natural Foods by Nancy Appleton, PhD
Healthy Healing by Linda Page, PhD, ND
Let's Play Doctor by J.D.Wallach, DVM, ND
Bragg Healthy Lifestyle by Paul C. Bragg, ND, PhD and Patricia Bragg, ND, PhD
Excitotoxins (The Taste That Kills) by Russell L. Blaylock, MD
The Super Anti-Oxidants by James F. Balch, MD
Nutrition & Physical Degeneration by Weston A. Price, DDS
Health in the 21st Century/Will Doctors Survive by Francisco Contreras, MD
Common Sense Health & Healing by Richard Schulze, ND
Patient Heal Thyself by Jordan Rubin, NMD, CNC
Immune Restoration Handbook (2nd edition) by Mark Konlee/ Conrad LeBeau
Miracle Food Cures from the Bible by Reese Rubin

Herbs
The Healing Power of Herbs by Michael Murray ND
Herbally Yours by Penny Royal
The Herb Book by John Lust ND, DBM
The 21st Century Herb Hyssop (The Superior Healing Power) by Willie Southall PhD

Juicing
Juice for Life by Sherry Calbom and Maureen Keane

Kinesiology

The Body Electric by Robert O. Becker
*Warning, the Electricity Around You May Be Hazardous to
Your Health* by Ellen Sugarman

Menopause
Before the Change by Ann Louise Gittleman
Natural Hormone Replacement Therapy for Women Over 45 by
    Jonathan Wright MD

Mercury Toxicity
It's All in Your Head by Hal Huggins DDS
Reversing Chronic Disease by Tom Warren
*Beyond Amalgam: The Hidden Health Hazard Posed by
Jawbone Cavitations* by Susan Stockton

Mental Health
Brain Recovery.com by David Perlmutter MD

Multiple Sclerosis
Solving the MS Mystery by Hal Huggins DDS

Vaccines
*The Sanctity of Human Blood: Vaccination Is Not
    Immunization* by Tim O'Shea

INDEX

F

Q

T

U

ENDNOTES

1   Mayo Clinic Staff. Metabolic Syndrome. http://www.mayoclinic. org/diseases-conditions/metabolic-syndrome/home/ovc-20197517 (accessed 9-9-16).

2   Amanda Spake and Mary B. Marcus, "A Fat Nation: America's Supersize Diet is Fatter and Sweeter—and Deadlier," US News and World Report, 8–19–02, Vol. 133, Is. 7, p. 40–47.

3   Ibid.

4   Ibid.

5   www.pbs.org, "Frontline: Diet Wars: Interview: Marion Nestle," (accessed 11–11–07).

6   www.who.int, "World Health Organization Assesses the World's Health Systems," (accessed 8-24-16).

7   www.cdc.gov/nchs, "Deaths," (accessed 7-4-16).

8   www.diabetes.org, "All About Diabetes, Diabetes Statistics," (accessed 6-7-16).

9   www.usatoday.com, "An Overweight America Comes With a Hefty Price Tag," (accessed 11-4-15).

10 www.nih.gov, Word on Health, 6–02, "Childhood Obesity on the Rise" (accessed 6-9-16).

11 S. Jay Olshansky, "A Potential Decline in Life Expectancy in the United States in the 21st Century," New England Journal of Medicine, Vol. 352:1138–1145, 3–17–05.

12 Eric Schlosser, Fast Food Nation: The Dark Side of the All American Meal, (NY: Perennial Press, 2002), p.3.

13 www.gcnm.com, "Why I Regularly Cleanse My Colon and Detoxify My Body," Global College of Natural Medicine, (accessed 6-8-16).

14 www.asu.edu, "Soft Drink Pouring Rights: Marketing Empty Calories," (accesses 10-6-15).

15 www.coloncancer.about.com, "Colorectal Cancer Death Statistics for the U.S.," (accessed 9–20–07).

16 www.cbsnews.com, "Americans Eat Themselves to Death," (accessed 6-9-16).

17 www.medscape.com, "Osteoporosis: Epidemiology, Diagnosis, and Treatment," (accessed 2-28-16).

18 www.nof.org, (accessed 5-5-16).

19 Ibid.

20 L. Steingrimsdottir, "Relationship Between Serum Parathyroid Hormone Levels, Vitamin D Sufficiency, and Calcium Intake," JAMA, 2005; 294: 2336–2341, (accessed 8-8-16).

21 Elizabeth Baker, The Uncook Book, (WA: Drelwood Press, 2000), p. 45.

22 Katherine Tucker, *et al.*, "Colas, But Not Other Carbonated Beverages are Associated with Low Bone Mineral Density in Older Women: The Framingham Osteoporosis Study," American Journal of Clinical Nutrition, 84, 10–1-06, p. 936–942.

23 www.cspinet.org, "Soft Drinks Undermining Americans' Health," (accessed 7-9-16).

24 Ibid.

25 www.cspinet.org, "Soft Drinks Undermining Americans' Health," (accessed 7-7-16).

26 Carol Simontacchi, The Crazy Makers, (NY: Jerry P. Tarcher/Putman, 2000), p. 20.

27 www.nof.org., "Bone is Living Tissue That Responds to Exercise by Becoming Stronger," (accessed 9-18-16).

28 Yu-Xiao Yang, et.al., "Long-term Proton Pump Inhibitor Therapy and Risk of Hip Fracture," JAMA, 2006, 296: 2947–2953, (accessed 11-1-15).

29   www.drugdigest.org1, "Proton Pump Inhibitors - Drug Comparisons - Compare Drugs,"(accessed 4-6-16).

30   James and Phyllis Balch, Prescription for Nutritional Healing, (NY: PenguinPutman Inc, 2000), p. 188.

31   www.med.umich.edu, "Green Tea Compound May be a Therapy for People with Rheumatoid Arthritis University of Michigan Study Finds," 4–30–07, (accessed 5-30-16).

32   Op. Cit., Balch, p. 506.

33   Jean Carper, Food–Your Miracle Medicine, (NY: Harper Perennial, 1993), p. 277–278.

34   Alzheimer's Foundation of America. http://www.alzfdn.org/AboutAlzheimers/statistics.html

35 |FCO|Hyperlinkwww.census.gov,"Aging Population,"|FCC| (accessed 1-11-16).

36   David Perlmutter, BrainRecovery.com, (The Perlmutter Health Center, 2000), p. 105.

37   Russell Blaylock, Excitotoxins, Health and Nutrition Secrets That Can Change Your life, (Albuquerque: Health Press, 2002).

38   Op. Cit., Balch, p. 169.

39   www.teens.drugabuse.gov, "Facts on Drugs: the Brain and Addiction," (accessed 1-10-15).

40   José Luchsinger and Richard Mayeux, "Cardiovascular Risk Factors and Alzheimer's Disease," Current Atherosclerosis Reports, Vol. 6, No.4, 7–04, p. 261–266.

41   Op. Cit., Carper, p. 288–290.

42   www.web-books.com, "Medicine, Cardiovascular, Heart Attack," (accessed 6-9-16).

43   The American Heart Association. https://www.heart.org/idc/groups/ahamah-public/@wcm/@sop/@smd/documents/downloadable/ucm_480086.pdf

44   www.emedicinehealth.com, "High Blood Pressure Article," (accessed 9-9-16).

45   www.emedicinehealth.com, "High Blood Pressure," (accessed 4-16-15).

46   www.cnn.com, "Evidence Suggests That Giving Blood Has Health Benefits," (accessed 11-16-15).

47   L. Bazzano, et.al., "Dietary Fiber Intake and Reduced Risk of Coronary Heart Disease in US Men and Women," Arch Intern Med, 2003, vol. 163, p. 1897–1904.

48   G. Fraser, "A Possible Protective Effect of Nut Consumption on Risk of Coronary Heart Disease," Arch Intern Med, 1992; 152, p. 1416–23.

49   Joan Bartlett, et.al., "Rebounding on a Mini-Trampoline: Implications for Physical Fitness and Coronary Risk Factors," Journal of Cardiopulmonary Rehabilitation, 1990, 10, p. 401–408.

50   Op. Cit., Balch, p. 129–130.

51   Ibid., p. 389.

52   Jonathan Wright, Dr. Wright's Guide to Healing with Nutrition, (PA: Rodale Press, 1984), p. 51–52.

53   JR Thornton, "Diet and Gall Stones: Effects of Refined and Unrefined Carbohydrate Diets on Bile Cholesterol Saturation and Bile Acid Metabolism," Gut., 1983 January; 24(1): 2–6.

54   Brenda Watson and Leonard Smith, Gut Solutions, (FL: Renew Life Press and Information Services, 2003), p. 184.

55   Gayla and John Kirschmann, Nutrition Almanac, Fourth Edition, (NY: McGraw-Hill, 1996), p. 260.

56   www.time.com, "Cut Out the Liver," Time Fit Nation Archive, 4–16–51, (accessed 6-30-16).

57   Op. Cit., Balch, p. 68.

58   Linda Page, Linda Pages' Healthy Healing, (CA: Healthy Healing Publications, 2001), p. 428.

59   www.endocrineweb.com, "How Your Thyroid Works," (accessed 7-8-16).

60 John Ott, Health and Light: The Effects of Natural and Artificial Light on Man and Other Living Things, (NY: Devin-Adair Publishing, 1972).

61 Daniel L. Roberts, Age Related Macular Degeneration, (NY: Marlowe & Co., 2006), p. 49.

62 Paul Jacques, "Long-term Vitamin C Supplement Use and Prevalence of Early Age-related Lens Opacities," Am J Clin Nutr, 1997, Oct, 66:4, 911–6.

63 www.glaucoma.org, "What is glaucoma?" (accessed 12-12-15).

64 www.lifescience.com, "Moving Your Eyes Improves Memory Study Suggests,"(accessed 6-8-16).

65 Norman Krinsky, et al., "Biologic Mechanisms of the Protective Role of Lutein and Zeaxanthin in the Eye," Annual Review of Nutrition, 7–03, Volume 23, p. 173–201.

66 www.ars.usda.gov, "Science Links Nutrition and Eye Health," (accessed 12-27-15).

67 www.ezinearticles.com, "Exercise Your Face to Look Healthier & Younger," (accessed 5-18-16).

68 In person interview with Elizabeth Baker on 1-6-02.

69 Paavo Airola, How To Get Well, (AZ: Health Plus Publishers, 1974), p. 244.

70 Op. Cit., Balch, p. 532.

71 David Reuben, The Save Your Life Diet, (NY: Bantam Books, 1968), p.8.

72 Spoken at a Get Healthy, America! seminar, Miami, 10–13.

73 Op. Cit., Wright, p. 52–53.

74 www.medicationsense.com, "The Magnesium Solution for Migraine Headaches," (accessed 1-29-16).

75 Op. Cit., Carper, p. 436.

76 Ibid, p. 336.

77 Ibid, p. 176.

78   Op. Cit., Balch, p. 154.

79   www.aafp.org, "American Family Physician, Allergy Testing," (accessed 12-12-15).

80   www.delta-clinic.com, "Applied Kinesiology," (accessed 9-1-16).

81   Op. Cit., Baker, p. 33–34.

82   www.emedicine.com, "Psychogenic Nonepileptic Seizures," (accessed 10-10-15).

83   www.wikepedia.org, (accessed 4-24-16).

84   www.wikipedia.org, "Hypoglycemia," (accessed 12-27-15).

85   www.westonaprice.org, "Soft Drinks: America's Other Drinking Problem," (accessed 10–5-07).

86   www.diabetes.org, "All About Diabetes", (accessed 1-5-16).

87   Op. Cit., Blaylock, p. 222.

88   Ibid p. 223.

89   Ibid p. 224.

90   Ibid p. 224.

91   John Tobe, Margarine, The Plastic Fat and Your Heart Attack, (Ontario: The Provoker Press, 1960), p. 8.

92   www.wikipedia.org, "Interesterified Fat," (accessed 2-28-16).

93   www.Starbulletin.com, "Midwesterners are Stocking Up on Kimchee," (accessed 11-5-15).

94   www.japanesefood.about.com, "Natto and Nattokinase", (accessed 8-8-16).

95   www.kitchenproject.com, "History of Sauerkraut," (accessed 5-30-16).

96   www.medicalnewstoday.com, "Can Broccoli Sprouts, Cabbage, Ginkgo Biloba and Garlic Prevent Cancer? Apparently Yes," (accessed 11–11–07).

97   Op. Cit., Schlosser, p. 90.

98   R. Tuttle, "Effect of Altered Breakfast Habits on Physiologic Response," J Appl Physio, 1949; 1: 545–559.

99 Roger J. Williams, Nutrition Against Disease, (NY: Pitman Publishing, 1971).

100 Gary Null, Get Healthy Now! p. 47.

101 G.M. Briggs and Doris Calloway. Nutrition and Physical Fitness, 11th Edition, (NY: Holt, Rinehart and Winston, 1988), p.12.

102 Elizabeth Baker, Unbelievably Easy Sprouting, (WA: Drelwood Publications, 2007), p 1.

103 Ibid, p. 29.

104 www.brassica.com, "Bio: Dr. Paul Talalay, M.D," (accessed 3-30-16).

105 Megumi Murashima, et.al., "Phase 1 Study of Multiple Biomarkers for Metabolism and Oxidative Stress After One-Week Intake of Broccoli Spouts," BioFactors, 2014; 22, p. 271–275.

106 Op. Cit., Balch, p. 80.

107 Anne Wigmore, Why Suffer: How I Overcame Illness and Pain Naturally, (NY:Avery Publshing Group, 1985).

108 Eydie Mae, How I Conquered Cancer Naturally, (CA: Production House, 1975), p.90.

109 www.acgraceco.com, "Why I Need Vitamin E," (accessed 4-4-16).

110 Ibid.

111 Op. Cit., Carper, p.207.

112 Op. Cit., Carper, p. 208.

113 www.StopAgingNow.com, Jean Carper Column "New Disease Fighters," 3-20-14.

114 www.medicalnewstoday.com, "Watercress: Anti-Cancer Super food," (accessed 10-23-15).

115 www.usaweekend.com, "EatSmart," (accessed 5-12-16).

116 Op. Cit., Carper, p.289–290.

117 www.livescience.com, "Zinc Improves Memory of 7th-Graders," The Associated Press, 4–26–05, (accessed 1-14-16).

118 Op. Cit., Carper, p. 176.

119 Ibid, p. 136.

120 www.news.nationalgeographic.com, "Pomegranate Juice Fights Heart Disease Study Says," (accessed 11-15-15).

121 www.red-raspberry.org, The Washington Red Raspberry Commission, (accessed 9-9-16).

122 Op. Cit., Carper, p. 460.

123 G. Fraser, "A Possible Protective Effect of Nut Consumption on Risk of Coronary Heart Disease," Archives of Internal Medicine, 1992, Vol. 152, p. 1416–1423.

124 Op. Cit., Carper, p. 80–81.

125 Ibid, p. 432.

126 www.Findarticles.com "Lutein: Not Just For Eyes–Benefits of Lutein in Green Leafy Vegetables in Cardiovascular Disease," (accessed 3-30-15).

127 American Thoracic Society Meeting, 5–01.

128 Michio Kushi, Diet for a Strong Heart, (NY: St. Martin's Press, 1985), p. 8.

129 Sheryl London, The Versatile Grain and The Elegant Bean, (NY: Simon & Schuster, 1992), p. 10.

130 Op. Cit., Schlosser, p. 7.

131 Ibid, p. 10.

132 Op. Cit., Blaylock, p. 33.

133 Ibid, p. 33.

134 Jay Gordon, Good Food Today, Great Kids Tomorrow, (CA: Michael Wiese Productions, 1994), p. 103.

135 Vicki Lansky, The Taming of the C.A.NDY Monster, (MN: Meadowbrook Press, 1978), p. 4.

136 Ibid, p. 6.

137 Ibid, p. 6.

138 Lendon Smith, Improving Your Child's Behavior Chemistry, (NY: Prentice Hall, 1976), p. 97.

139 Ibid, p. 97.

140 Ben Feingold, The Feingold Cookbook, (NY: Random House Inc., 1979), p. 5–7.

141 Ibid, p. 5–7.

142 First 20 years of Life Key to Cancer Risk, Reuters newspaper, quoting a study reported in the International Journal of Cancer, 4–22–02.

143 Op. Cit., Schlosser, p. 122.

144 www.johnrobbins.com, (accessed 4-16-16).

145 Michael Murray, Diabetes and Hypoglycemia, (CA: Prima Publishing, 1994), p. viii.

146 Harvey Diamond, You CAN Prevent Breast Cancer! (CA: Promotion Publishing, 1996), p. 68.

147 Ibid., p. 243.

148 Ibid., p. 237.

149 Marilyn Diamond, A New Way of Eating, (NY: Warner Communications, 1981), p. ix.

150 Op. Cit., Murray, p. vii.

151 Op. Cit., Kushi, p. 33.

152 Op. Cit., Diamond, p. 83–84.

153 Op. Cit., Gordon, p. 9.

154 Op. Cit., Diamond, p. 242.

155 Ibid., p. 8.

156 Op. Cit., Diamond, p. 95.

157 John Robbins, Reclaiming Your Health, (CA: H.J. Kramer, 1996), p. 3.

158 Op. Cit., Murray, p. viii.

159 Ibid, p. iii.

160 Sharon Yntema, Vegetarian Children, a Supportive Guide for Parents, (IL: Login Trade, 1995), p. 11.

161 Charles Attwood, Dr. Attwood's Low-Fat Prescription for Kids, (NY: Penguin Books, 1995), forward.

162 Op. Cit., Smith, p. 97.

163 Ibid, p. 92.

164 Op. Cit., Attwood, p. 48.

165 www.seattletimes.com, quote from the 1–7-03 issue of The Annuals of Internal Medicine.

166 Alice Water, Chef and owner of Chez Panisse restaurant in Berkeley, Calif. and a major contributor to the movement toward healthy modern American cooking.

167 Op. Cit., Attwood, p. 59.

168 Op. Cit., Attwood, p. 71.

169 Op. Cit., Gordon, p. 63.

170 Maureen Salaman, Where's the Beef? National Health Federation Convention (4-6-11).

171 www.organicconsumers.org, "Beef Hormones Linked to Premature Onset of Puberty & Breast Cancer," (accessed 12-4-15).

172 "What About Dairy?" EarthSave Newsletter, Summer, 2015.

173 Op. Cit., Gordon, p. 48.

174 Jeffrey Goettemoeller, Stevia Sweet Recipes, (IL: Vital Health Publishing, 1998), p. 6.

175 Harvey and Marilyn Diamond, Fit for Life II: Living Health (NY: Warner Books, 1987), p. 58.

176 Op. Cit., Attwood, introduction.

177 Op. Cit., Gordon, p. 96.

178 www.SeattleTimes.com, Quote from the 1-7-14 issue, The Annuls of Internal Medicine.

179 Op. Cit., Yntema, p. 43.

180 David and Rachelle Bronfman, CalciYUM!, (Ontario, Bromedia Inc., 1998), p. 82.

181 Nancy Sokol Green, Poisoning Our Children, (IL: Noble Press, 1991), p. 36.

182 Ibid.

183 Ibid.

184 Ibid.

185 Ibid.

186 Ellouise Carroll, A Study of the Knowledge and Practices of Mothers in America Regarding Nutrition 2003, p. 8.

187 www.americanpregnancy.org, "Mercury Levels in Fish,"(accessed 11-2-14).

188 San Diego Family Magazine, "Cancer and Breastfeeding Connection," San Diego, CA., 5–13, p. 98.

189 Op. Cit., Balch, p. 85.

190 Michael Murray, The Healing Power of Herbs, (CA: Prima Publishing, 1992), p. 1.

191 Phyllis Balch, Prescription for Herbal Medicine, (NY: Avery Press, 2012), p. 33.

192 S. Visudhiphan, "The Relationship Between High Fibrinolytic Activity and Daily Capsicum Ingestion in Thais," American Journal of Clinical Nutrition, 1982; 35: 1452–58.

193 Elizabeth Baker, spoken at a Get Healthy, America! seminar in FL, 8–03.

194 R. Shama, "Effect Of Fenugreek Seeds on Blood Glucose and Serum Lipids in Type I Diabetes," European Journal of Clinical Nutrition, Apr; 44(4):301–6.2013.

195 E.S. Johnson et.al., "Efficacy of Feverfew as Prophylactic Treatment of Migraine," Br Med J (Clin Res Ed), 1985, Aug 31;291(6495):569–73.

196 www.query.nytimes.com, "Read it and Steep," The New York Times, 1–19–03, (accessed 11-1-15).

197 Op. Cit., Murray, p. 161.

198 H. Woelk, "Benefits and Risks of the Hypericum Extract," Journal of Geriatric Psychiatry and Neurology, 7 (suppl): S34–38, 1994.

199 www.medicine.arizona.edu, "Turmeric Prevents Experimental Rheumatoid Arthritis and Bone Loss," (accessed 2-2-16).

200 Op. Cit., Carper, p. 399.

201 R.J. Lemire, "Neural Tube Defects," JAMA, 1988, Jan 22–29; 259(4): 558–62.

202 Op. Cit., Kirschmann, p. 63.

203 Op. Cit., Balch, p. 25.

204 B. Freidman-Graves, et al., "Manganese Balance and Clinical Observations in Young Men Fed Manganese Deficient Diet," Journal of Nutrition, 1987; 117: 133–134.

205 www.sciencenews.org, 5-3-03, Vol. 163, No. 18, (accessed 4-1-16).

206 Personal Journals of Elizabeth Baker, 10–1-04.

207 Bernard Jensen, Tissue Cleansing Through Bowel Management, (CA: The Jensen Publishing Enterprises 1981).

208 Robert O. and Shelly R. Young, Sick and Tired?, (UT: Woodland Publishing, 2001), p. 68.

209 www.med.nyu.edu, Global Institute for Alternative Medicine, quote from Ann Lousie Gittleman, (accessed 5-28-15).

210 Op. Cit., Young, p. 68.

211 O.M. Amin, "Seasonal Prevalence of Intestinal Parasites in the United States During 2000," Am. J. Trop. Med. Hygiene., 66(6), 2002, p. 799–803.

212 Ealine Sihera, 10 Easy Steps to Growing Old Disgracefully, (UK: Anser Publishing, 2014), p. 176.

213 F. Batmanghelidj, Your Body's Many Cries for Water, (VA: Global Health Solutions, 1997).